Atlas of
Ultrasound-Guided
Regional Anesthesia

Atlas of
Ultrasound-Guided
Regional Anesthesia

Andrew T. Gray, MD, PhD
Professor of Clinical Anesthesia
Department of Anesthesia and Perioperative Care
University of California, San Francisco School of Medicine
Staff Anesthesiologist
San Francisco General Hospital
San Francisco, California

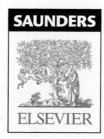

SAUNDERS

ELSEVIER

SAUNDERS
ELSEVIER

1600 John F. Kennedy Boulevard
Suite 1800
Philadelphia, PA 19103-2899

ATLAS OF ULTRASOUND-GUIDED REGIONAL ANESTHESIA ISBN 978-1-4377-0581-2

NOTICE

Knowledge and best practice in this field are constantly changing. As new research and experience broaden our knowledge, changes in practice, treatment and drug therapy may become necessary or appropriate. Readers are advised to check the most current information provided (i) on procedures featured or (ii) by the manufacturer of each product to be administered, to verify the recommended dose or formula, the method and duration of administration, and contraindications. It is the responsibility of the practitioner, relying on his or her own experience and knowledge of the patient, to make diagnoses, to determine dosages and the best treatment for each individual patient, and to take all appropriate safety precautions. To the fullest extent of the law, neither the Publisher nor the Author assumes any liability for any injury and/or damage to persons or property arising out of or related to any use of the material contained in this book.

The Publisher

Library of Congress Cataloging-in-Publication Data

Gray, Andrew T.
    Atlas of ultrasound-guided regional anesthesia / Andrew T. Gray.—1st ed.
        p. ; cm.
    Includes bibliographical references.
    ISBN 978-1-4377-0581-2
    1. Conduction anesthesia—Atlases.   2. Ultrasonic imaging—Atlases.   I. Title.
    [DNLM: 1. Anesthesia, Conduction.   2. Ultrasonography, Interventional. WO 300 G778a 2010]
    RD84.G73   2010
    617.9'640222—dc22

                                                                2009032809

Executive Publisher: Natasha Andjelkovic
Publishing Services Manager: Tina Rebane
Senior Project Manager: Amy L. Cannon
Senior Design Manager: Steven Stave
Multimedia Producer: Dan Martinez

Printed in China

Last digit is the print number: 9 8 7 6 5 4 3 2 1

To all the great writers in my family, especially MG.

ATG

PREFACE

For years I have spent my weekend afternoons reviewing footage of ultrasound-guided regional blocks. The vast majority of this footage is not worth saving, but what remains are the highlights and lowlights of my clinical practice in striking detail.

I make no apologies for using high-quality sonograms in *Atlas of Ultrasound-Guided Regional Anesthesia*. I feel that these images best illustrate the procedures and are easiest to learn from. Although the sonograms may not reflect all types of clinical imaging used today, imaging will continue to improve, and in the future, even more structural details will be evident. Good imaging is something to strive for because good imaging allows procedures to be safe and effective.

The images are intended to give the reader a specific idea of what to look for during regional anesthesia procedures and should prove helpful for people with a wide variety of backgrounds and clinical skills. Enough information is provided to enable the reader to understand and interpret the clinical ultrasound imaging of normal anatomy and its common variations. Limitations and artifacts also are discussed.

Special thanks to Drs. Robin Stackhouse and Susan Yoo who worked on recording the external photographs and Drs. Holger Baumann and Xiaokui Ma for providing some of the high-quality images. I also would like to thank the anesthesia workroom technical staff and Serafin Estrada at San Francisco General Hospital who helped me work on this project.

ANDREW T. GRAY, MD, PhD
August 2009

Contents

Section III Upper Extremity Blocks

Section IV Lower Extremity Blocks

Section V Trunk Blocks

Section VI Head and Neck Blocks

Section VII Safety Issues

SECTION I

Introduction to Ultrasound Imaging

CHAPTER 1

ULTRASOUND

Ultrasound waves are high-frequency sound waves generated in specific frequency ranges and sent through tissues.[1] How sound waves penetrate a tissue depends in large part on the range of the frequency produced. Lower frequencies penetrate deeper than high frequencies. The frequencies for clinical imaging (1-50 MHz) are well above the upper limit of normal human hearing (15-20 KHz). Wave motion transports energy and momentum from one point in space to another without transport of matter. In mechanical waves (e.g., water waves, waves on a string, and sound waves), energy and momentum are transported by means of disturbance in the medium because the medium has elastic properties. Any wave in which the disturbance is parallel to the direction of propagation is a longitudinal wave. Sound waves are longitudinal waves of compression and rarefaction of a medium such as air or soft tissue. *Compression* refers to high-pressure zones, and *rarefaction* refers to low-pressure zones (these zones alternate in position).

As the sound passes through tissues, it is absorbed, reflected, or allowed to pass through, depending on the echodensity of the tissue. Substances with high water content (e.g., blood, cerebrospinal fluid) conduct sound very well and reflect very poorly and thus are termed *echolucent*. Because they reflect very little of the sound, they appear as dark areas. Substances low in water content or high in materials that are poor sound conductors (e.g., air, bone) reflect almost all the sound and appear very bright. Substances with sound conduction properties between these extremes appear darker to lighter, depending on the amount of wave energy they reflect.

Reference

1. Aldrich JE. Basic physics of ultrasound imaging. *Crit Care Med.* 2007;35:S131-S137.

CHAPTER 2

SPEED OF SOUND

The speed of sound is determined by properties of the medium in which it propagates. The sound velocity equals $\sqrt{(B/\text{rho})}$, where B equals the bulk modulus, and *rho* equals density. The bulk modulus is proportional to stiffness. Thus, stiffness (change in shape) and wave speed are related. Density (weight per unit volume) and wave speed are inversely related. The speed of sound in a given medium is essentially independent of frequency.

Because the velocity of sound in soft tissue is 1540 m/sec, 13 microseconds elapse for each centimeter of tissue the sound wave must travel (the back-and-forth time of flight). Speed of sound artifacts relate to both time of flight considerations and refraction that occurs at the interface of tissues with different speeds of sound.[1-3]

References

1. Scanlan KA. Sonographic artifacts and their origins. *AJR Am J Roentgenol.* 1991;156:1267-1272.
2. Fornage BD. Sonographically guided core-needle biopsy of breast masses: the "bayonet artifact." *AJR Am J Roentgenol.* 1995;164:1022-1023.
3. Gray AT, Schafhalter-Zoppoth I. "Bayonet artifact" during ultrasound-guided transarterial axillary block. *Anesthesiology.* 2005;102:1291-1292.

Bayonet artifact

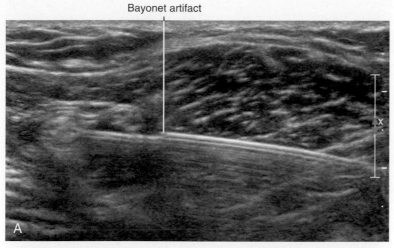

Bayonet artifact

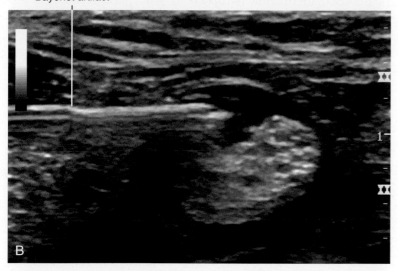

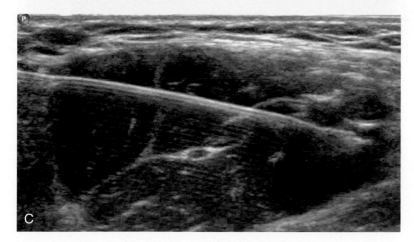

Figure 2-1. Bayonet artifacts during popliteal block (**A** and **B**). Because the speed of sound is not necessarily homogeneous in soft tissue, the needle can sometimes appear to bend, similar to a bayonet. Actual mechanical bending of the needle typically appears as gentle bowing of the needle (**C**).

CHAPTER 3

ATTENUATION

Attenuation is a decrease in wave amplitude as it travels through a medium. The attenuation of ultrasound in soft tissue is about 0.8 dB/(MHz-cm), indicating that the extent of attenuation depends on the distance traveled and the frequency of insonation. The units of the attenuation coefficient directly show the greater attenuation of high-frequency ultrasound beams. In soft tissue, 80% or more of the total attenuation is caused by absorption of the ultrasound wave, thereby generating heat.

Time gain compensation (TGC) adjusts for attenuation of an ultrasound beam as a function of depth. When TGC is properly adjusted, images of similar reflectors appear the same regardless of depth.

An acoustic shadow is said to exist when a localized object reflects or attenuates sound to impede transmission. Bone is a strong absorber of ultrasound waves. Therefore, shadowing occurs deep to bony structures ("bone shadow").

When a nonattenuating fluid (e.g., blood or injected local anesthetic) lies within an attenuating sound field (e.g., soft tissue), enhancement of echoes deep to the fluid occurs. This phenomenon, originally described as *posterior acoustic enhancement* (also called *increased through-transmission*), is due to lack of absorption of the sound waves by the fluid.[1] This attenuation artifact is a potential source of problems, especially during regional blocks where nerves are situated close to blood vessels.

Clinical Pearls

- In general, the highest frequency capable of adequate penetration to the depth of interest should be used for imaging.
- Decibels (dB) are a relative logarithmic measure of sound wave intensity.

Reference

1. Filly RA, Sommer FG, Minton MJ. Characterization of biological fluids by ultrasound and computed tomography. *Radiology.* 1980;134:167-171.

Ulna

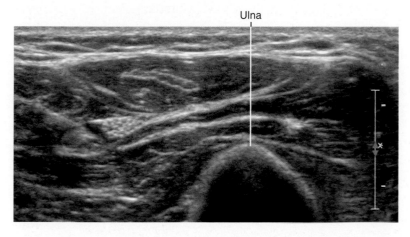

Figure 3-1. Acoustic shadowing by bone. In this sono-gram from the forearm, the acoustic shadowing by the ulna is evident. The bright cortical line of the surface of the bone is followed by extinction of the sound wave below.

CHAPTER 4

REFLECTION

Ultrasonography measures the amplitude of the return echo as a function of time.[1] Sound waves are reflected at the interface of tissues with different acoustic impedances. The acoustic impedance (kg/m^2/sec) is the product of the density (kg/m^3) and velocity (m/sec). The extent of reflection is governed by the reflection coefficient: $R = (Z1 - Z2)/(Z1 + Z2)$. If $Z1 = Z2$, there is no reflected wave.[2] Ultrasound characteristics of biologic tissue and interventional materials are summarized in Table 4-1.

Reflections off a smooth surface are called *specular*. If two specular reflectors are close to each other, reverberation within the sound field can result, displayed as parallel, equally spaced lines deep to the reflectors. Comet-tail artifact, which is a form of reverberation artifact, is caused by multiple internal reflections from a small, highly reflective interface.[3,4]

TABLE 4-1	Ultrasound Characteristics of Biologic Tissue and Interventional Materials		
SUBSTANCE	**VELOCITY (m/sec)**	**ATTENUATION (dB/[MHz-cm])**	**IMPEDANCE (MRayls × 10^{-6})**
Air	330	7.5	0.0001
Water	1480	0.0022	1.5
Soft tissue	1540	0.75	1.7
Blood	1575	0.15	1.6
Bone	4080	15	8
Stainless steel	5790	0.2	47

Data from Ziskin MC. Fundamental physics of ultrasound and its propagation in tissue. *Radiographics.* 1993;13:705-709; Ziskin MC, Thickman DI, Goldenberg NJ, et al. The comet tail artifact. *J Ultrasound Med.* 1982;1:1-7; Gawdzinska K. Investigation into the propagation of acoustic waves in metal. *Metalurgija.* 2005;44:125-128; Smith SW, Booi RC, Light ED, et al. Guidance of cardiac pacemaker leads using real time 3D ultrasound: feasibility studies. *Ultrason Imaging.* 2002;24:119-128.

Clinical Pearls

- The normal pleural line is thin and smooth, which generates a few comet-tail artifacts (between one and six artifacts per intercostal space scan). In the presence of parenchymal lung disease, the pleural line is irregular and thickened, generating many more comet-tail artifacts.[5]
- No comet-tail artifact is observed from the lung when pleural effusion is present.
- Hyperechoic reverberation artifacts are seen with metallic foreign bodies such as block needles.

References

1. Ziskin MC. Fundamental physics of ultrasound and its propagation in tissue. *Radiographics*. 1993;13:705-709.
2. Ziskin MC. Equation governing the transmission of ultrasound. *J Clin Ultrasound*. 1982;10:A21.
3. Ziskin MC, Thickman DI, Goldenberg NJ, et al. The comet tail artifact. *J Ultrasound Med*. 1982;1:1-7.
4. Thickman DI, Ziskin MC, Goldenberg NJ, Linder BE. Clinical manifestations of the comet tail artifact. *J Ultrasound Med*. 1983;2:225-230.
5. Reissig A, Kroegel C. Transthoracic sonography of diffuse parenchymal lung disease: the role of comet tail artifacts. *J Ultrasound Med*. 2003;22:173-180.

Reverberation artifact

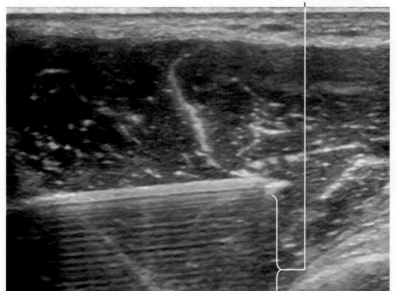

Figure 4-1. Reverberation artifact from a block needle placed nearly parallel to the active face of the transducer.

Comet-tail artifact

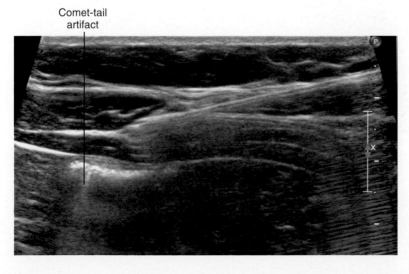

Figure 4-2. Comet-tail artifact from the peritoneum during rectus sheath block.

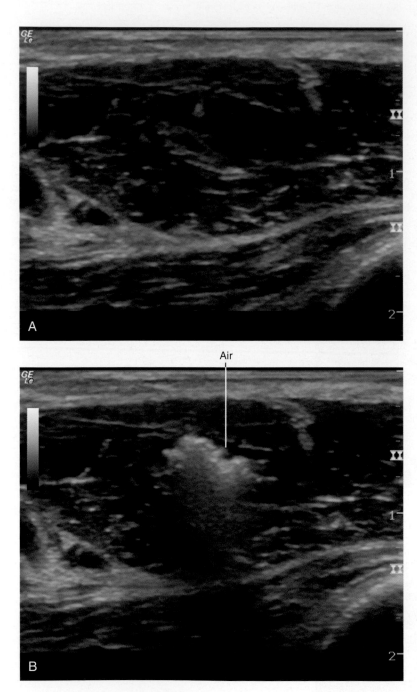

Air

Figure 4-3. A strong echo and acoustic shadowing are observed when air is inadvertently injected during musculocutaneous nerve block in the axilla. Sonograms before injection (**A**) and after injection (**B**) are shown.

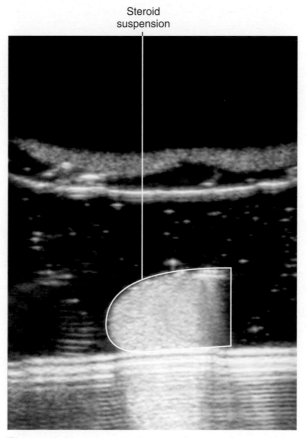

Figure 4-4. Acoustic properties of a steroid suspension. Although the local anesthetic injected for most regional blocks is anechoic, the particles of this steroid suspension are sufficiently large to produce a strong echo.

CHAPTER 5

BEAM WIDTH (SLICE THICKNESS)

Ultrasound systems assume all reflectors lie directly along the main axis of the ultrasound beam (i.e., the acoustic axis or central ray)[1]; however, ultrasound beams have a finite size. The out-of-plane beam width (slice thickness) can be measured with a diffuse scattering plane.[2] The plane is oriented at a 45-degree angle so that the displayed echoes are equal to the out-of-plane echoes. Ultrasound beams can be focused to reduce the out-of-plane beam width and thereby improve image quality.

References

1. Goldstein A, Madrazo BL. Slice-thickness artifacts in gray-scale ultrasound. *J Clin Ultrasound.* 1981;9:365-375.
2. Goldstein A. Slice thickness measurements. *J Ultrasound Med.* 1988;7:487-498.

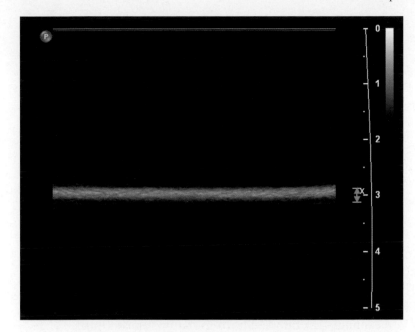

Figure 5-1. Out-of-plane slice thickness. Ultrasound scan of a diffuse scattering plane (a sheet of sandpaper).

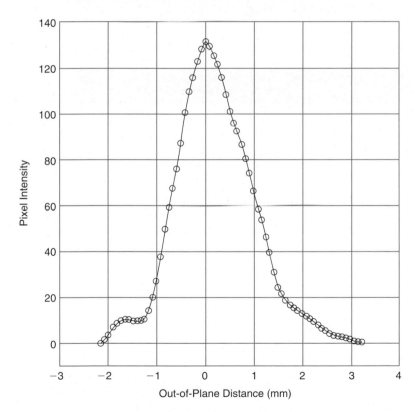

Figure 5-2. The beam profile is shown as a function of the distance from the central ray. Because needle diameters are substantially less than those of the slice plane, a strong relationship between needle diameter and visibility is expected.

CHAPTER 6

ANISOTROPY

Isotropic means equal in all directions. *Anisotropic* implies angle dependence. The latter term has been used to indicate the change in amplitude of received echoes from a structure when the angle of insonation is changed. Anisotropy is a discriminating feature between nerves and tendons. Tendons are more anisotropic than nerves, meaning that smaller changes in angle (about 2 degrees) alter the echoes from tendons than the changes in angle (about 10 degrees) that alter the echoes from nerves. The anisotropy of nerves also is important because during interventions, it can be challenging to maintain nerve visibility while manipulating the transducer to image the block needle.[1] With training, practitioners learn to naturally manipulate the transducer to fill in the received echoes from nerves. The amplitude of the received echoes from peripheral nerves is usually largest when the sound beam is perpendicular to the nerve path. Other structures, such as muscle, also exhibit anisotropy.[2]

Clinical Pearls

- Anisotropy means that the backscatter echoes from a specimen depend on the directional orientation within the sound field.
- Anisotropy can be quantified by specifying the transducer frequency and the decibel change in backscatter echoes with perpendicular and parallel orientation of the specimen.
- Nerves, tendons, and muscle all exhibit anisotropy. Of these structures, tendon echoes are the most sensitive to transducer manipulation.

References

1. Soong J, Schafhalter-Zoppoth I, Gray AT. The importance of transducer angle to ultrasound visibility of the femoral nerve. *Reg Anesth Pain Med*. 2005;30:505.
2. Rubin JM, Carson PL, Meyer CR. Anisotropic ultrasonic backscatter from the renal cortex. *Ultrasound Med Biol*. 1988;14:507-511.

Median nerve

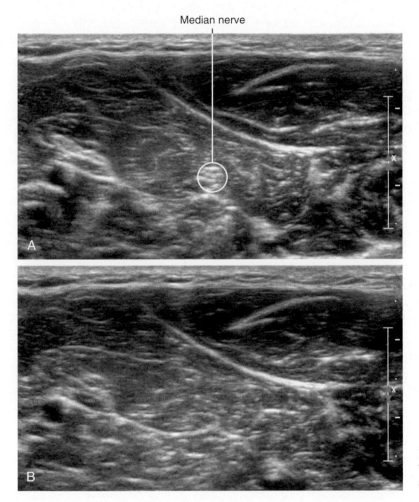

Figure 6-1. Anisotropy of the median nerve (**A** and **B**). With inclination of the transducer (tilting), the received echoes from the median nerve disappear.

CHAPTER 7

SPATIAL COMPOUND IMAGING

In conventional sonography, tissue is insonated from a single direction. Spatial compound imaging combines multiple lines of sight to form a single composite image at real-time frame rates. The ultrasound beam is steered by a different set of predetermined angles, typically within 20 degrees from the perpendicular.

One benefit of the use of spatial compound imaging is the reduction of angle-dependent artifacts (Table 7-1). *Speckle* is the granular appearance of a sonographic image that results from scattering of the ultrasound beam from small tissue reflectors. This speckle artifact results in the grainy appearance observed on sonograms, representing noise in the image. Improved image quality may be obtained by using spatial compound imaging, which can reduce speckle noise.

There is a central triangular region of overlap within the field of view where all angles mesh together for full compounding. The corners of the image receive only a subset of all the lines of sight; therefore, not all the benefits of spatial compounding are manifest. Some machines allow the stray lines of sight (those off the rectangular field of view) to form a trapezoidal image format. This is sometimes useful to view the approaching needle with in-plane technique.

Ultrasound imaging near bone may be improved by spatial compound imaging. This has relevance to imaging for some blocks (e.g., neuraxial, paravertebral, lumbar plexus, intercostals, sacroiliac joint). Although ultrasound waves cannot penetrate mature bone (even with low-frequency ultrasound), spatial compound imaging allows better definition of the bone surface.

Linear test tool images can be used to reveal the number of lines of sight used in spatial compound imaging. These images are generated with a smooth metal surface, such as that of a paper clip, solid metal stylet, or a U.S. nickel. Metal is used because it is relatively nonattenuating and yet produces an echo. Smooth metal is used so that the test tool does not damage the transducer. For these measurements, high receiver gain and a single focal zone near the surface are used. As long as the test tool contact is less than the receiver aperture, the width of the displayed echoes will not change.

TABLE 7-1	**Advantages and Disadvantages of Spatial Compound Imaging**
ADVANTAGES	**DISADVANTAGES**
Reduction of angle-dependent artifacts (e.g., posterior acoustic enhancement and speckle)	Frame averaging (persistence or motion blur effect)
Needle tip imaging	Limited angle effects (typically <20 degrees)
Nerve border definition	
Fascia contours	
Imaging around bone	
Wider field of view with stray lines of sight	

Clinical Pearls

- The use of spatial compound imaging can improve imaging of nerve borders and the block needle tip.
- One potential disadvantage of compound imaging is that needle reverberations occur over a broader range of angles and can prevent imaging of deeper structures.
- Compound imaging is being developed for both linear and curved arrays.
- Sliding the transducer along the known course of the nerve is a well-established technique to improve small nerve imaging. However, frame rate reduction that occurs with spatial compound imaging can cause problems with this technique.
- If compound imaging is not an advantage for a particular imaging situation, it can be turned off.

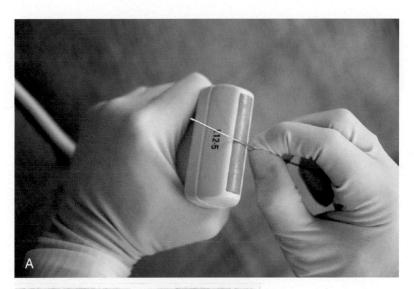

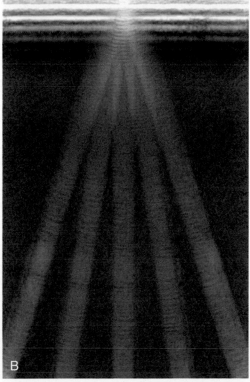

Figure 7-1. Spatial compound imaging. Some forms of ultrasound imaging use multiple lines of sight by electronically steering the beam to different angles. This sonogram was obtained by placing a linear array test tool (the solid metal stylet of a 17-gauge epidural needle) over the active face of the transducer to isolate a single element (**A** and **B**). The displayed test tool image consists of the receiver apertures of the transducer. In this case, five lines of sight are used to form a compound image.

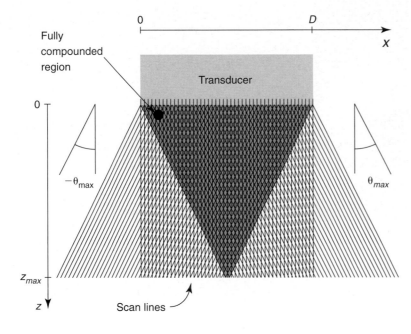

Figure 7-2. Conceptual illustration of transducer and associated scan lines for recording of three single-angle images. (Adapted from Jespersen SK, Wilhjelm JE, Sillesen H. In vitro spatial compound scanning for improved visualization of atherosclerosis. *Ultrasound Med Biol.* 2000;26:1357-1362.)

Doppler Imaging

The Doppler shift is the change in frequency of sound when the sound wave strikes a moving object. This means the frequency of the transmitted and reflected sound waves are not the same. Doppler shifts in clinical imaging are in the audible range (±10 KHz). Red blood cells are the primary reflectors that produce Doppler shifts. Ultrasound machines can color-encode the mean velocity (color Doppler), variance within the sample volume (variance Doppler), and power spectrum of the frequency shift (power Doppler).[1]

The optimal spectral Doppler angle is 30 to 60 degrees. Doppler angles greater than 60 degrees result in small Doppler shifts. Doppler angles less than 30 degrees result in loss of signal due to refraction.

Aliasing (incorrect or ambiguous estimation of the velocity) occurs when the velocity scale is set too small relative to the actual velocities. Wrap-around transition between positive and negative velocity on spectral Doppler tracings indicates aliasing; therefore, the peak velocities are off-scale and not accurately estimated. This occurs because the pulse repetition frequency is insufficiently low relative to the frequency of the Doppler signal (a consequence of the sampling or Nyquist theorem).

Color Doppler is traditionally shown with the Nyquist velocity limits. Color aliasing is displayed as reversed flow within laminar flow areas, with no intervening black stripe between them. With true flow reversal, the transition has an intervening black stripe, indicating no flow estimation. This narrow colorless area occurs because of the absence of a Doppler shift where flow is perpendicular to the angle of insonation.

Clinical Pearls

- Blood has a low ultrasound attenuation coefficient. Red blood cells are the primary reflectors within blood.
- In power Doppler, the gain threshold can be adjusted to the level at which there is no observed signal in bone.[2]
- In low-flow states (e.g., heart failure or atrial arrhythmias), aggregates of red blood cells can cause spontaneous contrast within blood vessels.

References

1. Bude RO, Rubin JM. Power Doppler sonography. *Radiology*. 1996;200:21-23.
2. Rubin JM. Musculoskeletal power Doppler. *Eur Radiol*. 1999;9(Suppl 3):S403-S406.

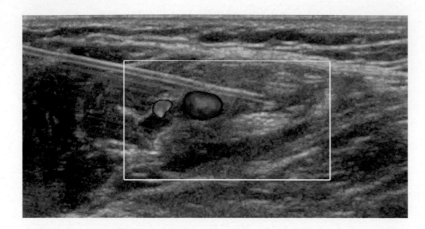

Figure 8-1. An example of color Doppler imaging during axillary block. A short-axis view of the neurovascular bundle is displayed.

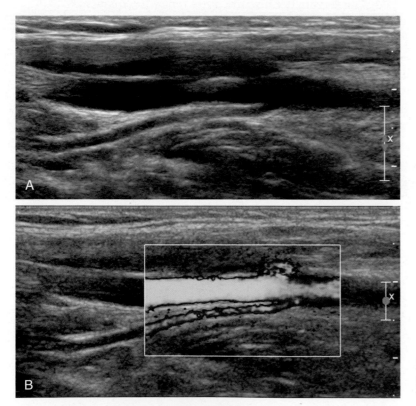

Figure 8-2. Long-axis view of the axillary artery and its profunda branch in conventional B-mode imaging (**A**) and with power Doppler (**B**).

CHAPTER 9

ULTRASOUND TRANSDUCERS

Ultrasound transducers consist of arrays of piezoelectric crystals that produce high-frequency sound waves in response to an electrical signal. These crystals interconvert electrical and mechanical energy, allowing for both transmission and reception of sound waves. The piezoelectric element vibrates to produce ultrasound. Piezoelectric crystals change shape under the influence of an electric field. The thickness of the crystal and the propagation speed within determine the frequency. With some transducers, the sonographer can select different crystals within the assembly to produce a different frequency.

The first ultrasound transducers were made using natural piezoelectric crystals (quartz, Rochelle salts, tourmaline). Modern transducers use synthetic crystals, such as PZT (lead zirconate titanate), which have high density, velocity, and acoustic impedance.

Linear arrays typically produce a rectangular image format. The piezoelectric crystals are arranged in a straight line. Curvilinear arrays produce images in sector format (that do not originate from a single point). The range of angles with curved arrays (typically, 0 60 degrees) is much larger than with beam steering for spatial compound imaging (typically, 0-20 degrees).

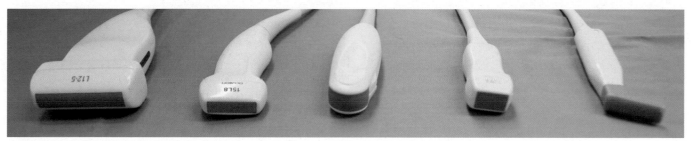

Figure 9-1. Ultrasound transducers for regional blocks. The photograph includes (*left to right*) broad linear, small footprint linear, curved, sector, and hockey-stick transducers.

CHAPTER 10

TRANSDUCER MANIPULATION

Nomenclature for transducer manipulation has been previously established.[1] Note that this nomenclature does not include specification of direction (e.g., rock back, rotate clockwise, tilt proximal). To control the transducer for interventions, the hands of the operator must be very close to the skin surface. The ulnar aspect of the transducer hand should rest on the skin of the patient.

Reference

1. AIUM Technical Bulletin. Transducer manipulation. American Institute of Ultrasound in Medicine. *J Ultrasound Med.* 1999;18:169-175.

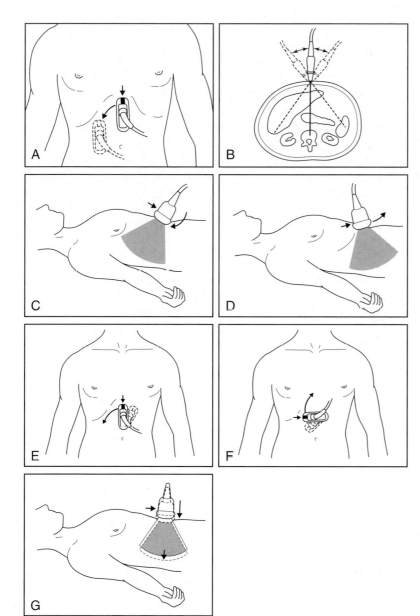

Figure 10-1. To optimally display anatomy for image presentation, the transducer must be manipulated. Transducer manipulation can be broken down into five basic movements: sliding (**A**), tilting (**B**), rocking (**C** and **D**), rotating (**E** and **F**), and compressing (**G**). Combining these movements allows for smooth scanning motion and anatomy visualization. (Adapted from AIUM Technical Bulletin. Transducer manipulation. American Institute of Ultrasound in Medicine. *J Ultrasound Med.* 1999;18: 169-175.)

CHAPTER 11

NEEDLE IMAGING

Needle tip visibility is critical to the success and safety of regional block interventions. It is imperative to identify the needle tip before advancing the needle. The cut on the bevel is the best identifier of the needle tip for a beveled needle. Partial line-ups (so that the needle tip is not within the plane of imaging but some of the needle shaft is) are a source of false reassurance with in-plane technique. A number of factors have been reported to influence needle tip visualization under clinical imaging conditions (Table 11-1).

Insertion Angle (Angle of Insonation)

Needle tip imaging is optimal when the needle is parallel to the active face of the transducer. The cleanest needle echo is from a conventional needle at or near parallel. One study found a linear correlation between angle of incidence (measured from 0-75 degrees) and the mean needle tip brightness.[1]

Needle Gauge

There are multiple advantages to using a large needle for regional block. Needles as large as 17 gauge have been used to improve needle tip visibility for regional blocks.[2] Alignment of a large needle is faster with in-plane technique. An additional advantage of a large needle is the ability to redirect the needle within the scan plane. A large needle tip can be used to displace structures (e.g., arteries or nerves) before advancing. The disadvantages of the large needle are patient discomfort and the consequences of unintended puncture (e.g., of vessels, nerves), which are typically worse. In addition, the soft tissue properties (tent and recoil) are

TABLE 11-1 **Factors Reported to Influence Needle Tip Visibility**

Angle of insonation

Needle gauge

Bevel orientation

Receiver gain

Needle motion and test injections

Echogenic modifications

Spatial compound imaging

more noticeable with large needles. With finer needle tips, the hand motion and needle tip motion are more closely matched, and it is easier to place a fine needle tip within a thin fascial plane.

Bevel Orientation

Needle bevel orientation is important for needle tip visibility (Table 11-2).[3] The bevel should be facing the transducer to enhance needle tip imaging.

Receiver Gain

The overall two-dimensional receiver gain should be reduced to improve visibility of the needle tip. However, a competing consideration is the visibility of other structures, such as the local anesthetic injection and blood vessels.

Needle Motion and Test Injections

Some clinicians move the needle slightly or use small-volume test injections (<1 mL) to improve the needle tip visibility.[4] Because regional anesthesia interventions are performed near reactive structures, if needle motion is used, it should be small and slow (avoid rapid jabbing motions, which may cause puncture or paresthesia).

Echogenic Modifications

McGahan roughened up the surface of needles with a No. 11 surgical blade to improve the needle tip visibility.[5] Historically, this was one of the first echogenic needle designs. When

TABLE 11-2	Influence of Bevel Orientation on Needle Tip Visibility		
ANGLE (DEGREES)	POOR	FAIR	GOOD
0	0.14	0.45	0.41
90	0.33	0.51	0.17
180	0.14	0.45	0.41
270	0.25	0.52	0.23

From Hopkins RE, Bradley M. In-vitro visualization of biopsy needles with ultrasound: a comparative study of standard and echogenic needles using an ultrasound phantom. *Clin Radiol.* 2001;56:499-502.

the angle of approach is more the 30 degrees, an echogenic needle is of benefit because the roughened surface sends echoes back to the transducer.[6]

Spatial Compound Imaging

With an increasing angle of incidence, the decrease in needle visibility is more pronounced for single-line ultrasound than for compound imaging. However, at angles of incidence of more than 30 degrees, the needle was barely visible with either method of imaging.[7]

Clinical Pearls

- Among specialized needles used for regional blocks, Hustead needle tips tend to have better ultrasound visibility.
- Side-port needles for regional block do not appear to exhibit isotropic diffraction, which has been reported to enhance the ultrasound visibility of similar needles.[8]
- Large-bore needles can be used as nerve retractors, pushing or pulling nerves out of the way of the advancing needle.
- Bevel orientation should be toward the nerve (so that the needle will pass the nerve rather than puncture it).
- When navigating the block needle between two nerves, the bevel should be rotated to face the closer of the two. This helps the block needle shoot the intervening gap and makes the closer nerve roll to the side as the needle is advanced. The same bevel orientation strategy can be used when placing the block needle between a nerve and an artery.

References

1. Bondestam S, Kreula J. Needle tip echogenicity: a study with real-time ultrasound. *Invest Radiol.* 1989;24:555-560.
2. Sandhu NS, Capan LM. Ultrasound-guided infraclavicular brachial plexus block. *Br J Anaesth.* 2002;89:254-259.
3. Hopkins RE, Bradley M. In-vitro visualization of biopsy needles with ultrasound: a comparative study of standard and echogenic needles using an ultrasound phantom. *Clin Radiol.* 2001;56:499-502.
4. Feller-Kopman D. Ultrasound-guided internal jugular access: a proposed standardized approach and implications for training and practice. *Chest.* 2007;132:302-309.
5. McGahan JP. Laboratory assessment of ultrasonic needle and catheter visualization. *J Ultrasound Med.* 1986;5:373-377.
6. Deam RK, Kluger R, Barrington MJ, McCutcheon CA. Investigation of a new echogenic needle for use with ultrasound peripheral nerve blocks. *Anaesth Intensive Care.* 2007;35:582-586.
7. Cohnen M, Saleh A, Luthen R, et al. Improvement of sonographic needle visibility in cirrhotic livers during transjugular intrahepatic portosystemic stent-shunt procedures with use of real-time compound imaging. *J Vasc Interv Radiol.* 2003;14:103-106.
8. Hurwitz SR, Nageotte MP. Amniocentesis needle with improved sonographic visibility. *Radiology.* 1989;171:576-577.

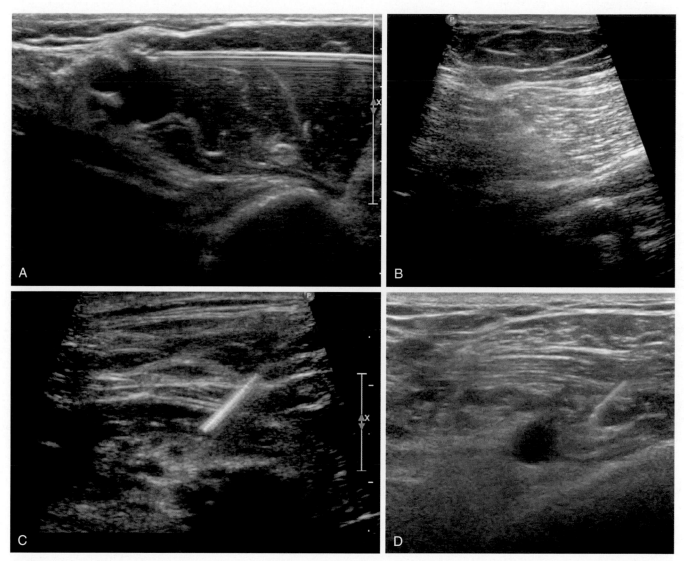

Figure 11-1. Influence of angle of insonation on needle tip visibility. When the needle is nearly parallel, the tip is easily identified (**A**). When the needle is at an angle, needle tip visibility is difficult (**B**). Echogenic needles can help improve needle tip visibility at steep angles under some clinical imaging conditions (**C** and **D**).

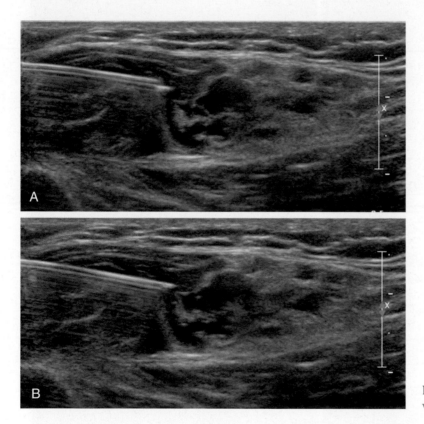

Figure 11-2. Influence of bevel orientation on needle tip visibility: bevel up (**A**) and bevel down (**B**).

CHAPTER 12

Approach Techniques

There are two basic approaches to ultrasound guidance. With the out-of-plane technique, the needle tip crosses the plane of imaging as an echogenic dot. With the in-plane approach, the entire tip and shaft of the advancing needle are visible.

Out-of-Plane Approach

There are several advantages to the out-of-plane approach to regional block (Table 12-1). This approach is most similar to traditional approaches to regional block guided by nerve stimulation or palpation. Therefore, the out-of-plane approach provides a natural transition from one form of guidance to another. The out-of-plane approach uses a shorter needle path than in-plane approaches. If short-axis views of the nerve are used, an out-of-plane approach results in catheter placement that is guided along the path of the nerve. One disadvantage of the out-of-plane approach is the extent of the unimaged needle path (structures that may lie short of or beyond the scan plane). If the needle tip crosses the scan plane without recognition, it can be advanced beyond the scan plane into undesired tissue.

In-Plane Approach

There are several advantages to the in-plane approach. It provides the most direct visualization of the needle tip and injection. The amount of unimaged needle path is typically small.

TABLE 12-1 Comparison of Out-of-Plane and In-Plane Approaches

APPROACH	ADVANTAGES	DISADVANTAGES
Out-of-plane (OOP)	Most similar to other approaches to regional block (nerve stimulation or palpation) Shorter needle path than with in-plane approaches Along the nerve path (catheters)	Unimaged needle path, crossing the plane of imaging without recognition
In-plane (IP)	Most direct visualization	Partial line-ups (creating a false sense of security when the needle tip is not correctly identified) Some unimaged needle path occurs with IP approach, but typically less than with OOP approach Longer paths and therefore more structures to cross with the block needle

The needle tip is visualized before advancement. One disadvantage is the long needle path, which results in more tissue for the needle to cross. Large-bore needles are often used with this approach to facilitate alignment. Partial line-ups (visualization of the needle shaft without visualization of the needle tip in the scan plane) create a false sense of security and therefore compromise safety of the technique.

External marks on the transducer can be used to guide needle placement for in-plane technique. However, the mechanical axis of the transducer and its acoustic axis are not always precisely aligned.[1]

Off-Line Markings

Off-line techniques involve external skin markings from ultrasound scans without imaging during needle placement. Changes in patient position, mobility of the skin, and dynamic changes with needle placement and injection limit the utility of this approach. The skin adjacent to the sides of the transducer can be marked. Alternatively, a paper clip or solid metal stylet (preferably with dull ends) can be used to create artifact within the field to mark the position of the object. For this technique, spatial compound imaging should be turned off to enhance the artifact.[2] The M-mode center line can be used to facilitate off-line markings in the center of the field.

Hand-on-needle provides better needle control for in-plane technique. This is important for blocks above the clavicle where the injection hand is stabilized. Hand-on-syringe provides the ability to control needle movement and injection by one operator.

Skill is probably more important than approach alone. There will probably never be a good study comparing the two approaches (out-of-plane versus in-plane) because of strong institutional biases regarding how to perform regional blocks.

By musculoskeletal convention, the long-axis images will be shown with the proximal side on the left and the distal side on the right. Long-axis views are useful for demonstrating longitudinal distributions of local anesthetic along the nerve path in one image. However, in clinical practice, it is usually easier to view the nerve in short axis and slide along the nerve path. Right-handed operators prefer a right-hand screen bias so that they can see their hands and display during the procedure.

References

1. Goldstein A, Parks JA, Osborne B. Visualization of B-scan transducer transverse cross-sectional beam patterns. *J Ultrasound Med.* 1982;1:23-35.
2. Gabriel H, Shulman L, Marko J, Nikolaidis P. Compound versus fundamental imaging in the detection of subdermal contraceptive implants. *J Ultrasound Med.* 2007;26:355-359.

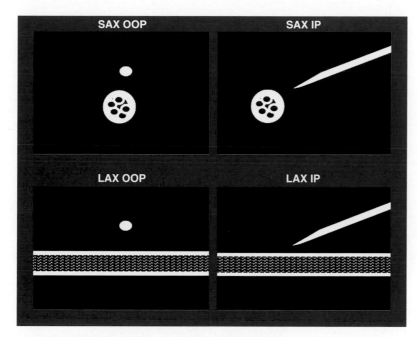

Figure 12-1. Schematic drawing of the short-axis and long-axis out-of-plane imaging (*left panels*), and short-axis and long-axis in-plane imaging (*right panels*). (Adapted from Gray AT. Ultrasound-guided regional anesthesia: current state of the art. *Anesthesiology.* 2006;104: 368-373.)

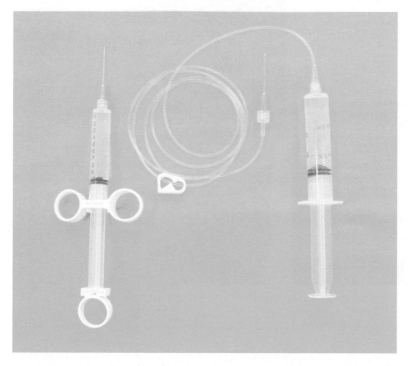

Figure 12-2. Set-up for regional block with hand-on-syringe or hand-on-needle approaches.

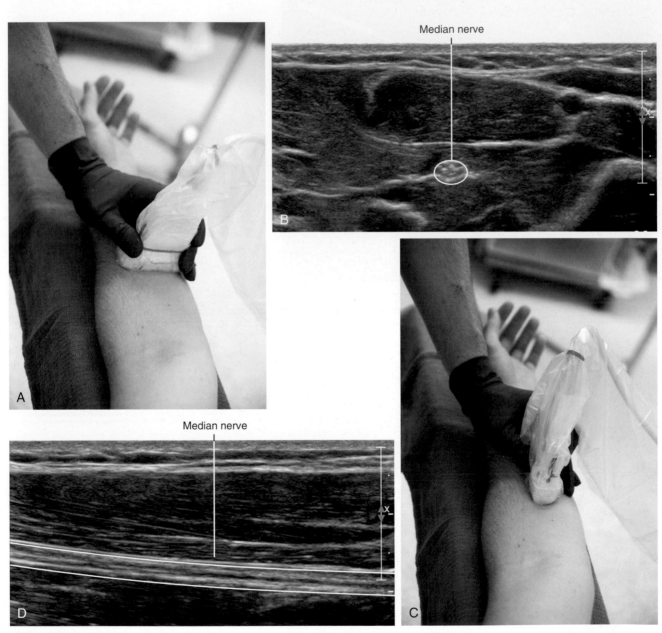

Figure 12-3. Median nerve viewed in short axis (**A** and **B**) and in long axis (**C** and **D**).

CHAPTER 13

SONOGRAPHIC SIGNS OF SUCCESSFUL INJECTIONS

It seems simple enough to state that successful drug injections for regional blockade should surround the peripheral nerve. However, recent studies have reported that the doughnut sign, previously considered the gold standard for success, has a positive predictive value of only 90% for producing surgical anesthesia.[1] It is therefore important to carefully consider multiple factors that constitute sonographic signs for success that can be evaluated after injection.

First, successful drug injections should clarify the nerve border. Most regional blocks are performed with nerves viewed in short axis to evaluate the circumferential distribution. If more that half of the nerve border is contacted by local anesthetic, it is unlikely there is an intervening fascial plane that will serve as a barrier to diffusion. Therefore, it is important that the injection round the corner of the nerve, so that there is demonstrated curvature of the injection.

Second, successful drug injections will track along the nerve. While the longitudinal distribution can be imaged with the nerve viewed in long axis, it is usually easier to slide the transducer along the nerve path with the nerve viewed in short axis (short-axis sliding assessment). If the local anesthetic truly tracks along the nerve, it will track along nerve divisions as well. This sign is especially useful for femoral and popliteal blocks because these block procedures are performed near points of nerve branching.

Third, peripheral nerves are often connected to adjacent structures, such as arteries or other peripheral nerves. Because they are covered in common connective tissue, successful injections should separate the connected structures. This is why practitioners often perform infraclavicular blocks or axillary blocks by placing the block needle tip between the axillary artery and the adjacent nerves. Understanding these connective tissue layers can provide a means of keeping the needle tip at a distance from the peripheral nerves.

Fourth, peripheral nerves are often more echogenic after injection of local anesthetic. This is because anechoic fluid has been injected into an attenuating sound field. This is not a perfect sign of success because anechoic fluid introduced anywhere between the nerve and the skin surface can cause this same effect.

Reference

1. Perlas A, Brull R, Chan VW, et al. Ultrasound guidance improves the success of sciatic nerve block at the popliteal fossa. *Reg Anesth Pain Med.* 2008;33.259-265.

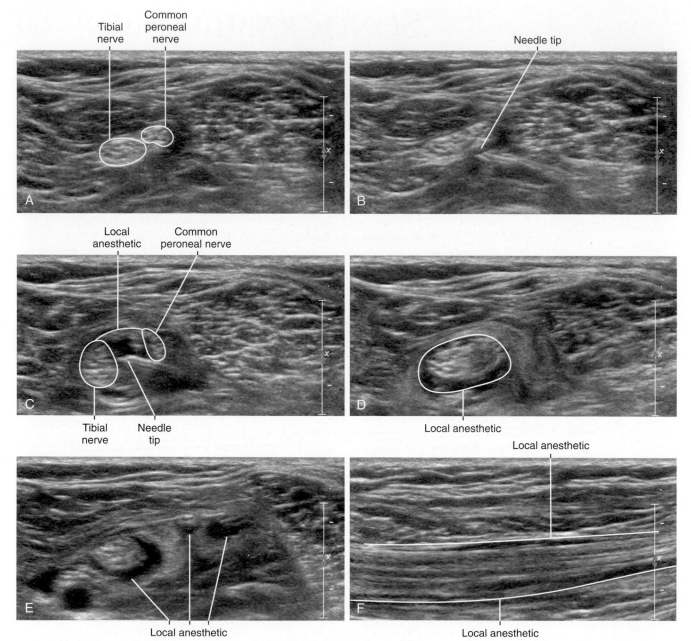

Figure 13-1. Image sequence showing successful sciatic nerve block in the popliteal fossa. The tibial and common peroneal contributions of the sciatic nerve are viewed in short axis before injection (**A**). An in-plane approach is demonstrated where the needle tip is placed between the tibial and common peroneal nerves (**B**). Local anesthetic is injected between the nerves (**C**). After injection, local anesthetic is distributed around the nerves (**D**), and tracks along nerve branches (**E**). A long-axis view also verifies the local anesthetic distribution along the sciatic nerve (**F**).

CHAPTER 14

Ultrasound-Guided Catheter Placement for Peripheral Nerve Blocks

Ultrasound-guided catheter placement is a complex procedure involving advanced manipulative skills of the operator.[1] Common procedures are ultrasound-guided interscalene, femoral, and popliteal catheters.[2] Out-of-plane approach is popular for peripheral nerve catheter insertion.[3]

The needle bevel should be turned so that the catheter slides along the nerve rather than around the nerve, in accordance with American Society of Regional Anesthesia guidelines.[4] A helically wound, metal-reinforced catheter can act as a spatially modulated wire.[5] Therefore, the ultrasound beam will be reflected back to the transducer regardless of the catheter orientation to improve visibility.

Long-axis in-plane approaches to peripheral nerve catheter placement have recently been reported.[6] The advantage is that the peripheral nerve, block needle, and catheter can all be viewed at the same time. However, it can be difficult to manipulate the transducer to maintain all three within the plane of imaging. Furthermore, because all three are constrained to lie in the same plane, care must be taken not to advance the needle and catheter into the nerve. Sciatic nerve catheters are particularly amenable to the long-axis in-plane approach if the patient can be placed in prone position. With this long-axis approach, the operator views directly across the patient for anatomic orientation of the ultrasound monitor.

References

1. Fredrickson MJ. Ultrasound assisted perineural catheter placement facilitated by a catheter introduction syringe. *Reg Anesth Pain Med.* 2007;32:370-371.
2. Swenson JD, Bay N, Loose E, et al. Outpatient management of continuous peripheral nerve catheters placed using ultrasound guidance: an experience in 620 patients. *Anesth Analg.* 2006;103:1436-1443.
3. Fredrickson MJ, Ball CM, Dalgleish AJ. Successful continuous interscalene analgesia for ambulatory shoulder surgery in a private practice setting. *Reg Anesth Pain Med.* 2008;33:122-128.
4. Borgeat A, Blumenthal S, Lambert M, et al. The feasibility and complications of the continuous popliteal nerve block: a 1001-case survey. *Anesth Analg.* 2006;103:229-233.
5. Trimmer WS, Vilkomerson D. A new wire phantom for accurate measurement of acoustical resolution. *Ultrason Imaging.* 5:87-93, 1983.
6. Koscielniak-Nielsen ZJ, Rasmussen H, Hesselbjerg L. Long-axis ultrasound imaging of the nerves and advancement of perineural catheters under direct vision: a preliminary report of four cases. *Reg Anesth Pain Med.* 33:477-482, 2008.

Catheter

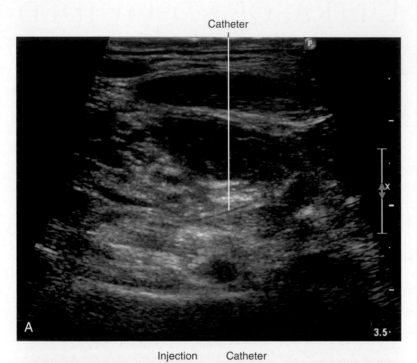

Injection   Catheter

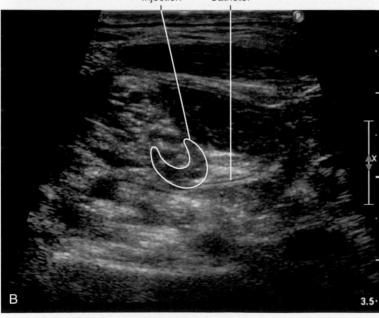

Figure 14-1. Ultrasound imaging of a peripheral nerve catheter in the interscalene groove. Sonograms are shown before (**A**) and after (**B**) injection of local anesthetic.

Needle tip

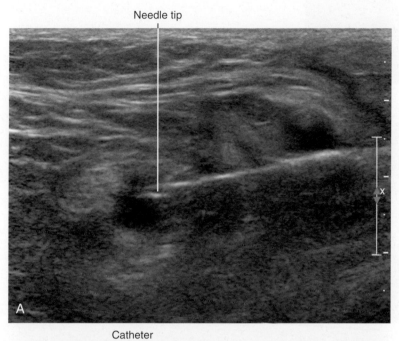

Catheter

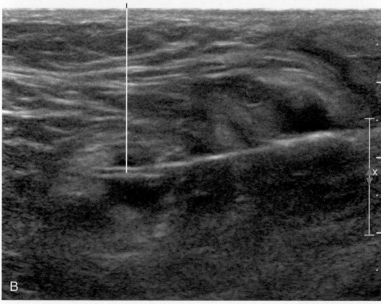

Figure 14-2. Advancement of a wire-reinforced catheter for popliteal block. Needle alignment before (**A**) and after (**B**) advancement of the catheter. A helically wound metal reinforced catheter can act as a spatially modulated wire. Therefore, the ultrasound beam will be reflected back to the transducer regardless of the catheter orientation to improve visibility.

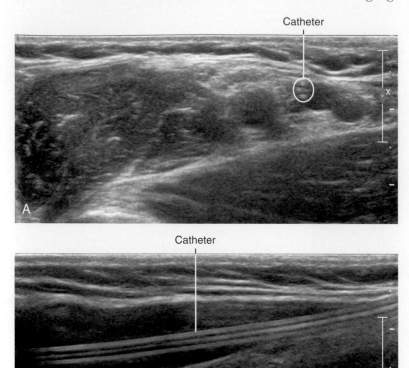

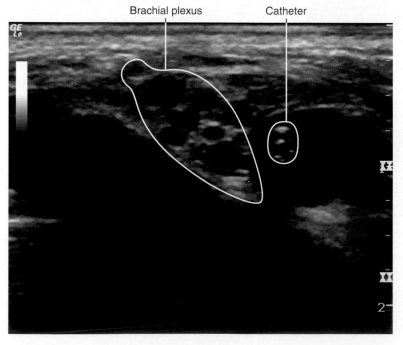

Figure 14-3. Peripherally inserted central catheter viewed in short axis (**A**) and long axis (**B**). This double-lumen catheter can appear similar to peripheral nerves in the axilla.

Figure 14-4. Multilumen catheter in the subclavian artery adjacent to the brachial plexus. The catheter and nerve have similar echotexture.

CHAPTER 15

THREE-DIMENSIONAL ULTRASOUND

There are now several reports of the use of three- or four-dimensional imaging to image nerves and guide peripheral blocks.[1-3] The complexity of the surrounding echoes in musculoskeletal tissue can make rendering clear three-dimensional images challenging. Injected anechoic fluid can improve the interface for three-dimensional imaging of the nerve surface. Rendered volumes are often shown with sepia coloring to improve contrast resolution.

One potential advantage of three-dimensional imaging is to avoid partial line-ups of the block needle that can occur with two-dimensional in-plane technique. Because line-up would not be necessary, performance time and accuracy of the procedure would benefit. One study found that the use of higher-dimensional imaging improved needle tip identification.[4] However, another study found that multiplanar reformatted displays improved needle conspicuity compared with volume-rendered displays.[5] Serious considerations for this developing technology balance obtaining more useful information with unnecessary distraction.

Manual acquisition of images by sliding the transducer at a constant velocity is difficult. Subsequent rendering of three-dimensional images is then done off-line. Another problem is that some probes used for three-dimensional imaging using automated sweeps of acquisition are large and bulky. The biggest benefit of three-dimensional imaging may be the detection of injections that would be out-of-plane with two-dimensional imaging (whether it is within a vessel or along a nerve).

Clinical Pearls

- Three-dimensional ultrasound has the same artifacts as two-dimensional imaging. Additional artifacts can arise from acquisition and rendering of three-dimensional images.
- Three-dimensional ultrasound may be useful for imaging the local anesthetic distribution when it tracks out of the plane of imaging for two-dimensional imaging.

References

1. Cash CJ, Sardesai AM, Berman LH, et al. Spatial mapping of the brachial plexus using three-dimensional ultrasound. *Br J Radiol.* 2005;78:1086-1094.
2. Feinglass NG, Clendenen SR, Torp KD, et al. Real-time three-dimensional ultrasound for continuous popliteal blockade: a case report and image description. *Anesth Analg.* 2007;105:272-274.

3. Foxall GL, Hardman JG, Bedforth NM. Three-dimensional, multiplanar, ultrasound-guided, radial nerve block. *Reg Anesth Pain Med.* 2007;32:516-521.
4. Won HJ, Han JK, Do KH, et al. Value of four-dimensional ultrasonography in ultrasonographically guided biopsy of hepatic masses. *J Ultrasound Med.* 2003;22:215-220.
5. Rose SC, Nelson TR, Deutsch R. Display of 3-dimensional ultrasonographic images for interventional procedures: volume-rendered versus multiplanar display. *J Ultrasound Med.* 2004;23:1465-1473.

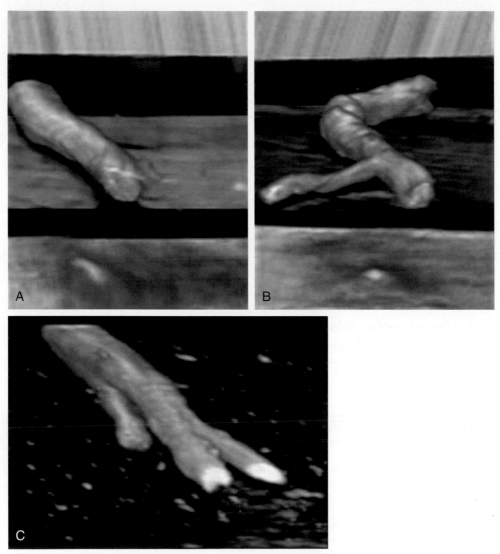

Figure 15-1. Excised ex vivo nerve specimen embedded in anechoic acoustic medium for three-dimensional imaging. A single nerve (**A**) and nerves with branching patterns (**B** and **C**) are displayed, demonstrating the echotexture of the nerve surface.

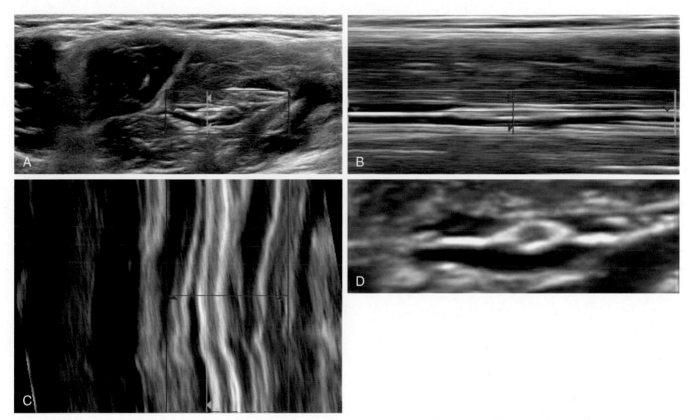

Figure 15-2. Clinical three-dimensional imaging of the musculocutaneous nerve and injection of local anesthetic. The nerve is seen in short-axis view (**A**), two long-axis views (**B** and **C**), and volume-rendered view (**D**).

Structures

CHAPTER 16

ANATOMIC STRUCTURES

Direct ultrasound visualization significantly improves the outcome of most techniques in regional anesthesia.[1] With the help of high-resolution ultrasonography, the anesthesiologist can directly visualize relevant structures for upper and lower extremity nerve blocks at all levels. Such direct visualization can improve the quality of nerve blocks and avoid complications. The benefits of directly visualizing targeted structures and monitoring the distribution of local anesthetic are significant. This ultrasound monitoring allows the anesthesiologist to reposition the block needle in the event of maldistribution of injected local anesthetic.

This section contains a brief overview of musculoskeletal imaging with ultrasound. There are several structures that are commonly imaged during regional blocks. Precise identification of these anatomic structures often involves tracking their course from start to end with ultrasound imaging.

Reference

1. Marhofer P, Greher M, Kapral S. Ultrasound guidance in regional anaesthesia. *Br J Anaesth*. 2005;94:7-17.

CHAPTER 17

SKIN AND SUBCUTANEOUS TISSUE

Normal skin (epidermis and dermis) is 1 to 4 mm thick and is uniformly hyperechoic. Subcutaneous tissue is hypoechoic with connective septa visible as streaks parallel or nearly parallel to the skin surface.

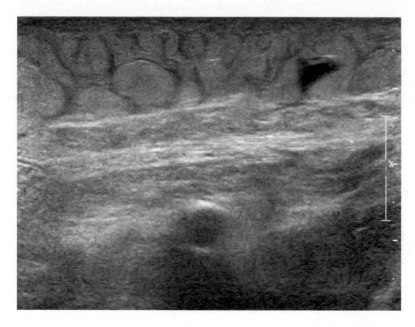

Figure 17-1. The river bed appearance to edema within subcutaneous tissue illustrating pathologic changes.

CHAPTER 18

PERIPHERAL NERVES

Peripheral nerves have a fascicular or "honeycomb" echotexture. This consists of the mixture of nerve fiber (hypoechoic) and connective tissue (hyperechoic) content within the nerve. Because there is little connective tissue within more central nerves (e.g., the cervical ventral rami of the brachial plexus), these nerves have a monofascicular or oligofascicular appearance on ultrasound scans.[1] Nerves that are surrounded by hypoechoic muscle are usually easier to visualize than nerves that are surrounded by hyperechoic fat because the nerve borders are more evident.

Peripheral nerves have a complex architecture. Nerves are like a plexus within themselves, with fascicles combining and recombining internally along the nerve path. Because of this intertwined network, the fascicle count will vary along the nerve path.[2] Nerve sections taken 2 mm apart can have different fascicular patterns.[2] The connective tissue content and fascicle count of peripheral nerves vary directly. That is, the amount of connective tissue is more abundant in multifascicular nerves.[3] The connective tissue within nerves protects the fascicles from injury. Therefore, monofascicular nerves are more vulnerable to damage.

Identification of nerve fascicles is the current basis of peripheral nerve imaging. With ultrasound, only a small subset of the total number of fascicles is imaged. In one study of ex vivo nerve specimens, only about one third the number of fascicles visible on light microscopy were visible on ultrasound scans.[4] It is difficult for imaging technologies to resolve thin collagenous boundaries between adjacent fascicles. For these reasons, fascicular discrimination is a standard by which to judge nerve imaging quality.

Nerves can be round, oval, or triangular. The shape can change along the nerve path or with heavy probe compression. Nerve fascicles are always round, and therefore monofascicular nerves are normally round. Despite changes in shape that may occur, nerves have a relatively constant cross-sectional area along their path.

High ultrasound frequencies (10-15 MHz) provide better resolution of nerve fascicles.[5] However, at lower frequencies (7-10 MHz), peripheral nerves are still visible as cordlike structures.[5] Commercial nerve imaging presets of imaging quality controls have been developed that enhance detection of nerve fascicles.

Short-axis sliding (sliding the transducer along the known nerve path with the nerve viewed in short axis) is a powerful technique not only to identify small nerves with ultrasound but also to assess the longitudinal distribution of local anesthetic along the nerve.

Among morphometric variables, the best correlate of nerve diameter is body height.[6] The best correlate of nerve visibility on ultrasound scans is the extremity size.[7]

Clinical Pearls

- When nerves cross a tight passage, they assume a more homogeneous hypoechoic appearance from tight packing of the nerve fascicles.[1]
- When scanning superficial nerves, it is best to apply a generous amount of acoustic coupling gel (as if applying toothpaste to a toothbrush) to provide some acoustic standoff.[8]
- Sliding along the known course of a peripheral nerve with the nerve viewed in short axis can be useful for determining the edges of the distribution.
- The easiest way to obtain a long-axis view of a peripheral nerve is to view it in short axis and rotate the probe while keeping the nerve in the center of the field of view.
- The outer band of collagen does not always produce a distinct echogenic nerve border. This can make long-axis assessments of local anesthetic distribution difficult.

References

1. Martinoli C, Bianchi S, Santacroce E, et al. Brachial plexus sonography: a technique for assessing the root level. *AJR Am J Roentgenol.* 2002;179:699-702.
2. Sunderland S. The anatomy and physiology of nerve injury. *Muscle Nerve.* 1990;13:771-784.
3. Sunderland S, Bradley KC. The cross-sectional area of peripheral nerve trunks devoted to nerve fibers. *Brain.* 1949;72:428-449.
4. Silvestri E, Martinoli C, Derchi LE, et al. Echotexture of peripheral nerves: correlation between US and histologic findings and criteria to differentiate tendons. *Radiology.* 1995;197:291-296.
5. Giovagnorio F, Martinoli C. Sonography of the cervical vagus nerve: normal appearance and abnormal findings. *AJR Am J Roentgenol.* 2001;176:745-749.
6. Heinemeyer O, Reimers CD. Ultrasound of radial, ulnar, median, and sciatic nerves in healthy subjects and patients with hereditary motor and sensory neuropathies. *Ultrasound Med Biol.* 1999;25:481-485.
7. Schwemmer U, Markus CK, Greim CA, et al. Sonographic imaging of the sciatic nerve division in the popliteal fossa. *Ultraschall Med.* 2005;26:496-500.
8. Thain LM, Downey DB. Sonography of peripheral nerves: technique, anatomy, and pathology. *Ultrasound Q.* 2002;18:225-245.

Cervical ventral
rami of the
brachial plexus

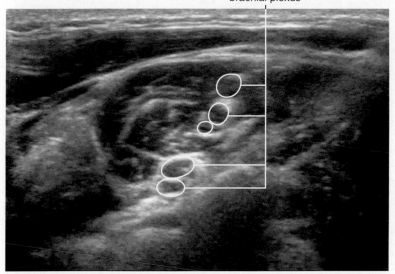

Figure 18-1. The cervical ventral rami of the brachial plexus viewed in short axis. This monofascicular echotexture is observed in more central nerves that contain little connective tissue.

Brachial plexus

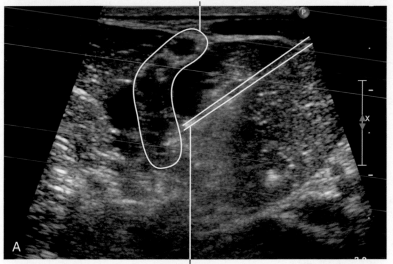

A

Needle tip

Local anesthetic

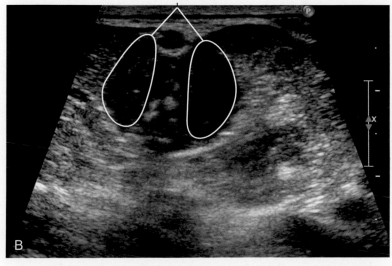

B

Figure 18-2. Interscalene block demonstrating monofascicular echotexture before (**A**) and after (**B**) injection of local anesthetic.

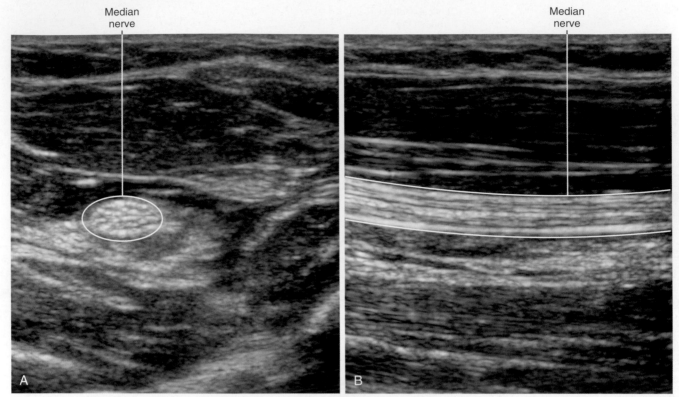

Median
nerve

Median
nerve

A

B

Figure 18-3. Median nerve in the forearm viewed in short axis (**A**) and long axis (**B**) demonstrating fascicular or honeycomb echotexture. These views were obtained after injection of local anesthetic around the nerve.

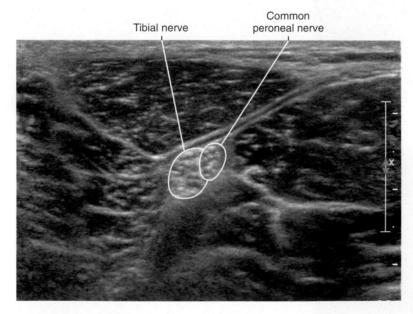

Tibial nerve

Common
peroneal nerve

Figure 18-4. Sciatic nerve in the thigh demonstrating echobright connective tissue content and compartmentalization into its tibial and common peroneal nerve components.

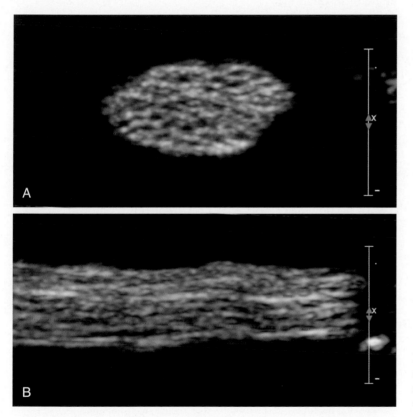

Figure 18-5. Excised ex vivo nerve specimen demonstrating fascicular echotexture in short-axis (**A**) and long-axis (**B**) views. Peripheral nerves viewed in long axis often exhibit parallel fascicles with coarse wavy echotexture.

CHAPTER 19

TENDONS

Tendons are the strong structures that connect muscle to bone. Their fibrillar echotexture (fiber-like, appearing as the fine hairs of a violin bow) results from parallel collagen bundles. Because of this ordered architecture, tendons are highly anisotropic, meaning that the received echoes are highly dependent on the angle of insonation.[1-3]

Tendons and nerves are both imaged during regional block procedures, and therefore some commentary regarding their discriminatory features is appropriate. Although the two structures can appear similar, tendons and nerves are primarily distinguished by tracing their course. Because tendons only form at the ends of muscle, changes in cross-sectional area along the course are substantial. For nerves, the cross-sectional area is relatively constant along the nerve path. In addition, the amplitudes of the received echoes from tendons are more sensitive to transducer inclination than nerves (tendons are more anisotropic than nerves). At high frequencies of insonation ($\geq$10 MHz), the fibrillar echotexture of tendons can be distinguished from the fascicular echotexture of nerves (Table 19-1).[4]

Tendons can have central or eccentric location within muscle depending on whether the muscle is bipennate or unipennate, respectively. Multipennate muscles have more than one tendon. Normal tendons are avascular with no flow detectable either on color-flow or power Doppler examinations.[5] Direct injections into tendons have been associated with tendon rupture.[6]

TABLE 19-1 **Characteristics of Nerves and Tendons That Can Be Identified With Ultrasound Imaging**

CHARACTERISTIC	NERVE	TENDON
Echotexture	Fascicular	Fibrillar
Elemental composition	Fascicles (coarse, thick, wavy, less numerous)	Fibrils (fine, thin, straight, more numerous)
Internal architecture	Plexiform (combine and divide)	Parallel fibrils
Cross-sectional area	Constant along nerve path	Forms at the ends of muscle
Overall shape	Round, oval, or triangular	Round, oval, or triangular; C or S
	Shape can change along path	Shape does not change along path
Branching	Yes	None
Anisotropy	Moderately sensitive	Highly sensitive
Adjacent vessels	Often	Infrequent
Border	Not as distinct	Distinct paratenon
Compressibility	More compressible	Less compressible

Some tendons are valuable landmarks of nerve position. For example, the ulnar nerve lies between the flexor carpi ulnaris (FCU) tendon and the ulnar artery in the medial forearm. As another example, the common peroneal nerve lies posterior to the conjoint tendon of the biceps femoris in the distal thigh near the knee crease. In the axilla, the neurovascular bundle lies anterior to the conjoint tendon of the latissimus dorsi and teres major.

Clinical Pearls

- The position of musculotendinous junctions is variable, making it difficult to identify tendons based on anatomic position alone.
- Tendons consist of a network of thin parallel and longitudinally oriented specular echoes that resemble fibrils. The septa consist of loose connective tissue with elastic fibers, vessels, and thin muscle fibers.
- Nerves typically have fewer and thicker echogenic lines than tendons.

References

1. Fornage BD. The hypoechoic normal tendon: a pitfall. *J Ultrasound Med*. 1987;6:19-22.
2. Crass JR, van de Vegte GL, Harkavy LA. Tendon echogenicity: ex vivo study. *Radiology*. 1988;167:499-501.
3. Connolly DJ, Berman L, McNally EG. The use of beam angulation to overcome anisotropy when viewing human tendon with high-frequency linear array ultrasound. *Br J Radiol*. 2001;74:183-185.
4. Silvestri E, Martinoli C, Derchi LE, et al. Echotexture of peripheral nerves: correlation between US and histologic findings and criteria to differentiate tendons. *Radiology*. 1995;197:291-296.
5. O'Connor PJ, Grainger AJ, Morgan SR, et al. Ultrasound assessment of tendons in asymptomatic volunteers: a study of reproducibility *Eur Radiol*. 2004;14:1968-1973.
6. Ford LT, DeBender J. Tendon rupture after local steroid injection. *South Med J*. 1979;72:827-830.

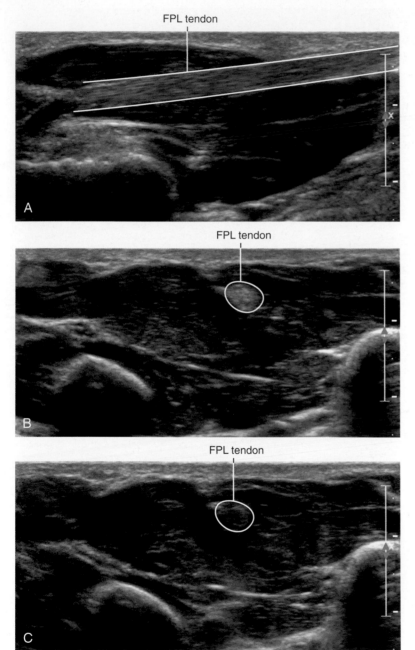

FPL tendon

FPL tendon

FPL tendon

Figure 19-1. The flexor pollicis longus (FPL) tendon in long-axis view (**A**) and short-axis view (**B**). If the transducer is tilted slightly, echoes from the tendon will disappear, thereby demonstrating anisotropy (**C**).

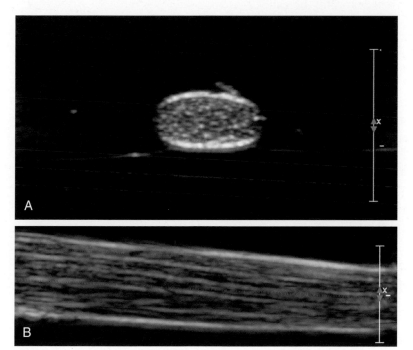

Figure 19-2. Excised ex vivo tendon specimen demonstrating fibrillar echotexture in short-axis (**A**) and long-axis (**B**) views.

20

PLANTARIS

The small plantaris muscle has a long, thin tendon that descends the leg deep to the medial head of the gastrocnemius. The plantaris tendon fuses with the medial side of the Achilles tendon. The plantaris tendon is absent in about 7% to 20% of individuals.[1] The plantaris muscle plantarflexes the foot and flexes the knee. The tendon of the plantaris muscle can have a similar appearance to the peripheral nerves of the leg. The plantaris tendon is to be distinguished from the sural nerve when scanning the calf.

Reference

1. Delgado GJ, Chung CB, Lektrakul N, et al. Tennis leg: clinical US study of 141 patients and anatomic investigation of four cadavers with MR imaging and US. *Radiology*. 2002;224:112-119.

Plantaris tendon

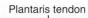

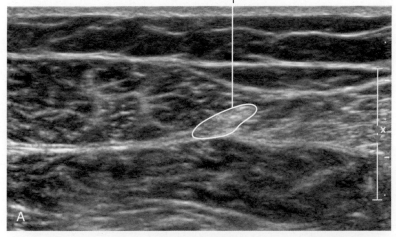

Plantaris tendon

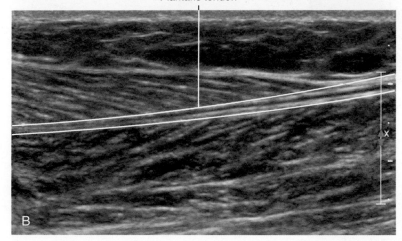

Figure 20-1. Plantaris tendon in short-axis (**A**) and long-axis (**B**) views. The tendon has a striking resemblance to a peripheral nerve. Unlike other tendons, the plantaris has a relatively uniform cross-sectional area. The plantaris tendon is deep to the medial head of the gastrocnemius, whereas the sural nerve is superficial. These images were obtained with the subject in prone position.

CHAPTER 21

ARTERIES

Visible pulsations from arteries are observed when compression is applied with the transducer to soft tissue. The amount of compression necessary for this depends on many variables, including the blood pressure, size and depth of the artery, and proximity of the artery to bone. Adjusting the amount of transducer compression to elicit visible pulsations is the fastest way to identify arteries. In some cases, it is necessary to apply Doppler. Arteries have thicker walls than veins and do not have valves. Almost every peripheral nerve has a long running path with accompanying artery or vein.

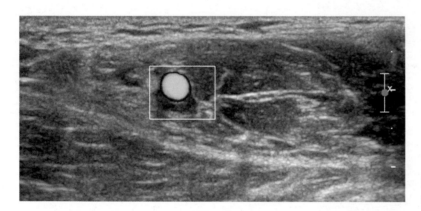

Figure 21-1. Short-axis view of the axillary artery in the axilla viewed with power Doppler.

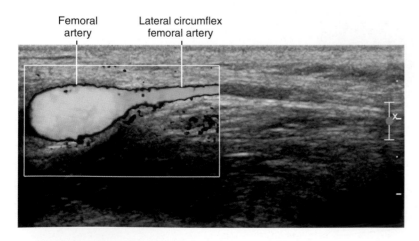

Figure 21-2. Power Doppler imaging of the femoral artery and lateral circumflex femoral artery. The lateral artery overlies the femoral nerve and is a potential site for bleeding complications.

Superficial cervical artery

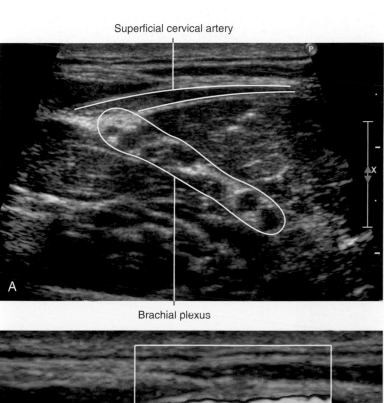

A

Brachial plexus

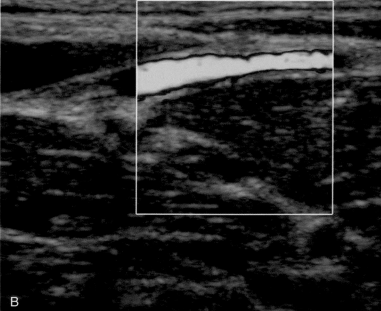

B

Figure 21-3. Superficial cervical artery is observed overlying the brachial plexus during interscalene block. **A,** B-mode sonogram. **B,** Power Doppler.

Femoral artery

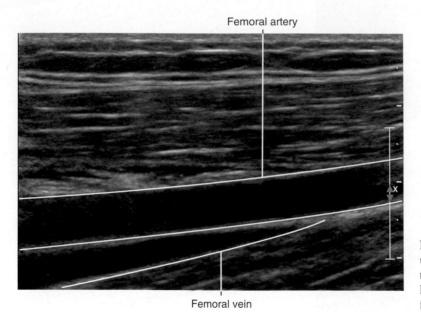

Femoral vein

Figure 21-4. Long-axis view of femoral artery running under the sartorius muscle in the mid-thigh proximal to the adductor canal. The femoral vein also is seen in long-axis view. The femoral artery servers as a landmark for saphenous nerve block in the mid-thigh.

CHAPTER 22

VEINS

Veins are easily compressed with the ultrasound transducer and have thin walls that are difficult to visualize. The vein shape is highly dependent on the amount of probe compression. Often, valves can be imaged inside the vein lumen. In contrast to the pulsatile flow of arteries, veins exhibit more continuous flow. Some degree of ACV waves and respiratory variation in flow may be present depending on how close the vein is to the thoracic cavity. Veins may have spontaneous contrast due to rouleaux formation of red blood cells in low-flow states such as congestive heart failure.[1] At the usual amount of probe compression for nerve imaging, the veins are not visible in the field because the vein walls are coapted.

Some veins travel with peripheral nerves within the subcutaneous tissue. The saphenous vein travels with the saphenous nerve in the medial leg. The small saphenous vein travels with the sural nerve in the lateral leg.

Reference

1. Machi J, Sigel B, Beitler JC, et al. Relation of in vivo blood flow to ultrasound echogenicity. *J Clin Ultrasound*. 1983;11:3-10.

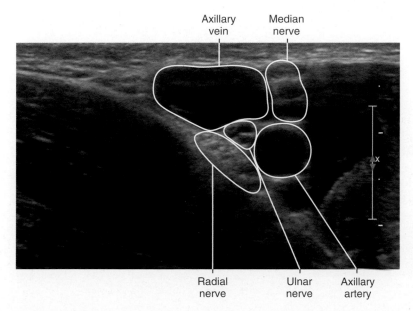

Figure 22-1. The axillary vein in the axilla. The ulnar nerve lies between the axillary artery and axillary vein in the axilla. The axillary vein can serve as an acoustic window for enhancing echoes from the ulnar nerve. In this sonogram, the ulnar nerve is shown in short-axis view deep to the axillary vein with light-touch imaging (no compression by the ultrasound transducer).

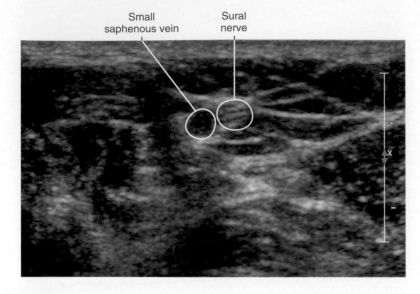

Small saphenous vein   Sural nerve

Figure 22-2. Short-axis view of the small saphenous vein and sural nerve within the subcutaneous tissue of the posterolateral calf. A calf tourniquet has been applied to distend the vein. Some veins serve as landmarks for nerve position.

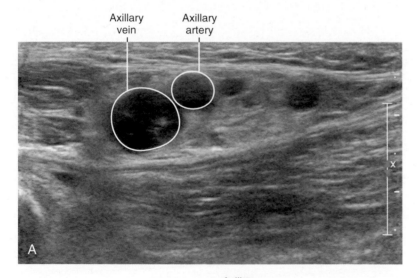

Axillary vein   Axillary artery

A

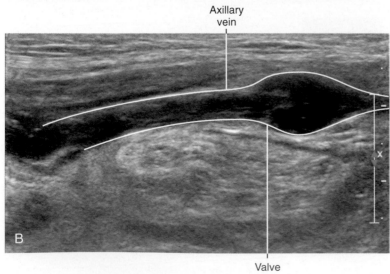

Axillary vein

B

Valve

Figure 22-3. Thrombosed (uncompressible) axillary vein in the axilla viewed in short axis (**A**) and long axis (**B**). A valve is present in the long-axis view.

23

BONES

The outer surface of cortical bone consists of dense fibrous connective tissue (the periosteum). There is a marked acoustic impedance mismatch between bone and soft tissue. This results in a bright line on ultrasound scans from reflection at the bone–soft tissue interface. Mature bone also is a great absorber of sound waves.[1] Acoustic shadowing occurs deep to the interface because of extinction of the sound wave.

Clinical Pearls

- Neuraxial scans of pediatric patients are superior to those of adults, in part because skeletal maturity does not occur until about 2 years of age from an acoustic standpoint.
- The thermal index of bone (TIB) is greater than thermal index of soft tissue (TIS) because of the substantial absorption of ultrasound.

Reference

1. Han S, Medige J, Davis J, et al. Ultrasound velocity and broadband attenuation as predictors of load-bearing capacities of human calcanei. *Calcif Tissue Int*. 1997;60:21-25.

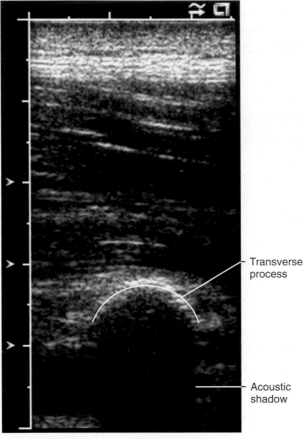

Transverse
process

Acoustic
shadow

Figure 23-1. Ultrasound appearance of bone, demonstrating a bright cortical line and acoustic shadowing. In this sonogram, a short-axis view of a transverse process is shown.

CHAPTER 24

PLEURA

The pleura is a strong reflector of ultrasound. Comet-tail artifact, indicating reverberation of sound waves, is observed deep to the pleural line on ultrasound scans.[1] Another characteristic feature of pleura with ultrasound imaging is "lung sliding."[2] The pleural line moves to and fro with ventilation. This motion is greatest at the base of the lung and least at the apex. Both comet-tail artifact and lung sliding are eliminated when pneumothorax is present.[3]

References

1. Thickman DI, Ziskin MC, Goldenberg NJ, Linder BE. Clinical manifestations of the comet tail artifact. *J Ultrasound Med.* 1983;2:225-230.
2. Lichtenstein DA, Menu Y. A bedside ultrasound sign ruling out pneumothorax in the critically ill: lung sliding. *Chest.* 1995;108:1345-1348.
3. Lichtenstein D, Meziere G, Biderman P, Gepner A: The comet-tail artifact: an ultrasound sign ruling out pneumothorax. *Intensive Care Med.* 1999;25:383-388.

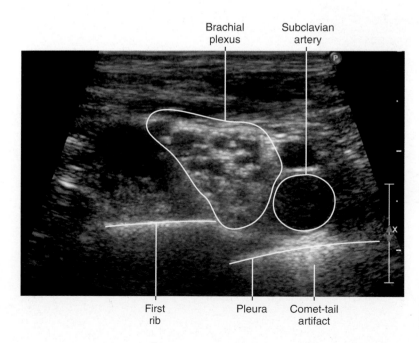

Figure 24-1. Comet-tail artifact observed deep to the pleural line during supraclavicular block of the brachial plexus.

CHAPTER 25

PERITONEUM

The peritoneum appears as a discrete, thin, smooth, single echogenic line deep to the abdominal wall.[1] Like pleura, peritoneum can produce a type of reverberation artifact known as *comet-tail artifact*.[2] Motion of the peritoneum and abdominal cavity contents ("gut sliding") can sometimes be appreciated.

References

1. Hanbidge AE, Lynch D, Wilson SR. Ultrasound of the peritoneum. *Radiographics*. 23:663-684, 2003.
2. Thickman DI, Ziskin MC, Goldenberg NJ, Linder BE. Clinical manifestations of the comet tail artifact. *J Ultrasound Med*. 2:225-230, 1983.

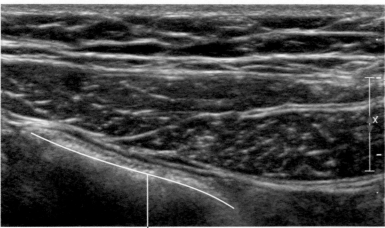

Peritoneum

Figure 25-1. Peritoneum deep to the abdominal wall muscles observed during rectus sheath block.

CHAPTER 26

LYMPH NODES

Normal lymph nodes are well-defined, oval structures containing an echogenic hilum and hypoechoic rim. Central vascularity can be demonstrated on Doppler scans (a hilar pattern of blood flow). Inguinal lymph nodes are frequently encountered during femoral nerve blocks. Lymph nodes are more numerous in young patients. Nodes involute with aging. Normal lymph nodes are small with well-defined borders.

Clinical Pearls

- Reactive lymph nodes are sometimes identified during regional blocks.
- Lymph nodes are small, oval, or reniform (bean shaped).
- Lymphatic vessels resemble veins in structure, but valves are more numerous in lymphatic vessels. The lymphatic vessels primarily contain lymphocytes (not erythrocytes).

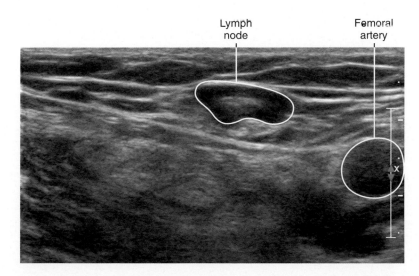

Figure 26-1. Ultrasound appearance of a lymph node in the inguinal region. This node was observed during femoral nerve block with ultrasound guidance.

Upper Extremity Blocks

CHAPTER 27

SUPRACLAVICULAR NERVE BLOCK

The supraclavicular nerve (SCN) is a branch of the superficial cervical plexus (see Fig. 58-1). It arises from the third and fourth cervical ventral rami and divides into three branches: medial, intermediate, and lateral. These branches are about 1 to 2 mm in diameter. The intermediate branch can in some cases be palpated over the mid-portion of the clavicle. The nerve has sensory fibers to the clavicle and shoulder, the chest wall to the level of the second rib, and the acromioclavicular and sternoclavicular joints.[1] The supraclavicular branches usually pass over the clavicle but in some cases can actually travel through the clavicle.[2,3] Block of the SCNs is useful for pain relief from shoulder or clavicle surgery.[4]

Suggested Technique

The traditional supraclavicular block of the brachial plexus is not considered adequate for shoulder surgery.[5] Sensory blockade of the supraclavicular and axillary nerves has slower onset for the traditional supraclavicular technique compared with the interscalene technique of brachial plexus anesthesia. However, ultrasound-guided infiltration of local anesthetic for SCN block can augment low interscalene or supraclavicular blocks for shoulder surgery. The SCN is typically located in the subcutaneous tissue over the brachial plexus near the clavicle. SCN block is generally performed after the brachial plexus block.

Clinical Pearls

- The incidence of the SCN branches piercing the clavicle is 1% to 4%.[6] In some of these cases, the bony foramina are large enough to be visible on chest radiographs.
- Interscalene blocks often result in SCN block because the local anesthetic tracks to C4 within the interscalene groove.[5] This is less likely or has slower onset with supraclavicular blocks of the brachial plexus. SCN blocks can be assessed along the skin surface over the clavicle.
- The SCNs further divide before piercing the platysma.

References

1. Mehta A, Birch R. Supraclavicular nerve injury: the neglected nerve? *Injury.* 1997;28:491-492.
2. Jelev L, Surchev L. Study of variant anatomical structures (bony canals, fibrous bands, and muscles) in relation to potential supraclavicular nerve entrapment. *Clin Anat.* 2007;20:278-285.
3. Jupiter JB, Leibman MI. Supraclavicular nerve entrapment due to clavicular fracture callus. *J Shoulder Elbow Surg.* 2007;16:e13-e14.
4. Choi DS, Atchabahian A, Brown AR. Cervical plexus block provides postoperative analgesia after clavicle surgery. *Anesth Analg.* 2005;100:1542-1543.
5. Lanz E, Theiss D, Jankovic D. The extent of blockade following various techniques of brachial plexus block. *Anesth Analg.* 1983;62:55-58.
6. Tubbs RS, Salter EG, Oakes WJ. Anomaly of the supraclavicular nerve: case report and review of the literature. *Clin Anat.* 2006;19:599-601.

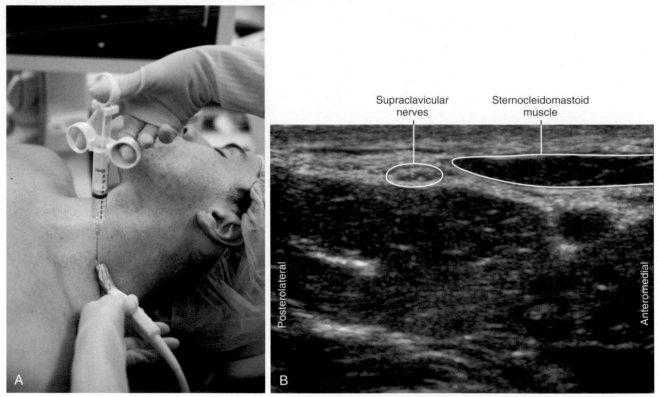

Figure 27-1. External photograph showing the approach to supraclavicular nerve block in the cervical region (**A**) and corresponding sonogram (**B**).

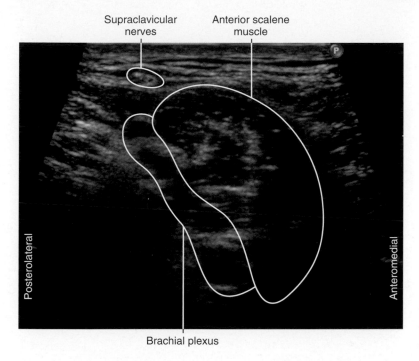

Supraclavicular nerves

Anterior scalene muscle

Posterolateral

Anteromedial

Brachial plexus

Figure 27-2. Short-axis view of the supraclavicular nerves before injection. The supraclavicular nerves are seen to lie superficial to the brachial plexus.

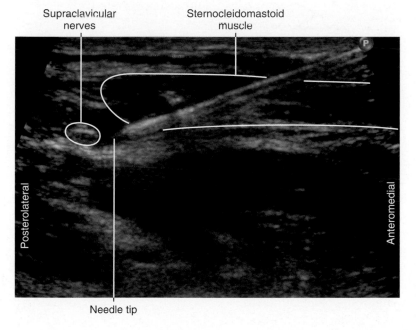

Supraclavicular nerves

Sternocleidomastoid muscle

Posterolateral

Anteromedial

Needle tip

Figure 27-3. Short-axis in-plane approach to block of the supraclavicular nerves of the cervical plexus. The block needle tip approaches from the medial side through the sternocleidomastoid muscle.

CHAPTER 28

INTERSCALENE AND SUPRACLAVICULAR BLOCKS

The first use of ultrasound to guide regional block was for brachial plexus block above the clavicle.[1] These pioneers used an off-line Doppler technique to mark the position of the subclavian artery as a surrogate landmark of the brachial plexus. Although today there may be many criticisms of this technique, their results were impressive: a 98% success rate with no complications.

Ultrasound imaging blurs the distinction between interscalene and supraclavicular blocks. If the brachial plexus is seen stacked between the anterior and middle scalene muscles, the block is generally referred to as an *interscalene block*. If the brachial plexus is seen as a compact group of nerves lying superior and lateral to the subclavian artery, the approach is generally referred to as a *supraclavicular block*. Because this distinction can be subtle, both blocks will be treated together.

Variations in brachial plexus anatomy with respect to the scalene muscles are common. The cephalad components of the plexus (in particular, the C5 and C6 ventral rami) often pass over or through the anterior scalene muscle. This may pose a problem for nerve stimulation–based approaches to brachial plexus blocks above the clavicle. The incidence of scalene muscle anomalies is similar for sonography of volunteers and in cadaveric dissections, suggesting that ultrasound can accurately detect these anomalies.[2]

Cervical ribs are relatively uncommon, occurring in about 0.5% of the population.[3,4] Most cervical ribs are partial (incomplete) and therefore will not pose a problem. However, if the cervical rib is sufficiently large, transducer manipulation can be difficult, and acoustic shadowing by the bone will obscure imaging of the brachial plexus.

Suggested Technique

The monofascicular ventral rami of the brachial plexus are hypoechoic and therefore can be difficult to identify between the scalene muscles. The ventral rami can be similar to blood vessels in their ultrasound appearance. The brachial plexus lies deep to the tapering posterolateral edge of the sternocleidomastoid in the neck.

The best nerve visibility is usually near the first rib because the brachial plexus is compact and lateral to the subclavian artery. The plexus contains more connective tissue moving from interscalene to supraclavicular views, resulting in more hyperechoic echotexture. To obtain a good supraclavicular view with the subclavian artery in true short axis, the imaging plane must face caudally to look down at the brachial plexus (not posteriorly). Brachial plexus imaging in the supraclavicular region is most consistent and can be used to trace the plexus back to the interscalene groove. Perform the block where the imaging is most reliable.

The semi-sitting (beach-chair) position helps comfort the patient, lowers the arm by gravity, and brings the plane of imaging closer to the plane of the display. The head-of-bed elevation should be about 45 degrees. The patient's head turns to the opposite side from the block. The operator stands either at the head of the bed or at the side of the bed, depending on the side of the block and the handedness of the operator.

Working room is limited above the clavicle, and therefore a compact transducer is favored. A small curved or small linear (20- to 25-mm footprint) transducer is preferred. The compact transducer can be rocked back to improve needle visibility. Broad linear probes are more difficult to rock than narrow linear or curved transducers for this procedure. The ulnar aspects of both hands of the operator are placed on the patient for the best control of the needle and transducer.

A short (50 mm), broad (21 gauge) echogenic needle is used for optimal control and visibility. Hand on needle (not hand on syringe) is recommended for better needle control. A medial to lateral in-plane needle path heads away from pleura.

Most authors recommend a multiple injection technique to ensure complete plexus anesthesia. With this approach, the initial aim of the needle is deep (under the more caudal elements of the plexus) so that the brachial plexus rises closer to the skin surface with the injection of local anesthetic. This makes the subsequent needle passes easier to perform. The needle tip should be positioned between the components of the brachial plexus for injection within the interscalene groove.[5] Inferior trunk sparing occurs less often with this multiple injection ultrasound technique compared with nerve stimulation–based approaches to interscalene block.[6]

The anatomy of the posterior triangle of the neck is complex. Nerves close to the brachial plexus, and therefore potentially in the needle path, include the phrenic nerve, dorsal scapular nerve, and spinal accessory nerve. The phrenic nerve lies medial to the brachial plexus and travels over the anterior scalene muscle toward the midline as it descends into the chest. The dorsal scapular nerve is a branch of the brachial plexus that is often observed lateral to the brachial plexus within the middle scalene muscle. The spinal accessory nerve is difficult to image but lies lateral to the brachial plexus within the posterior triangle of the neck.[7]

The number of visualized components of the brachial plexus (five ventral rami, three trunks, and six divisions) will vary with the angle of the transducer and its position in the neck. A mixture of these elements is possible within a given field of view. Sparing of the superficial cervical plexus and intercostobrachial nerves can occur.

A sterile transparent dressing (Tegaderm; 3M Health Care, St. Paul, Minn) can be used to cover the hockey-stick transducer for better external visualization of the probe position and therefore easier line-ups.[8] For this technique, the adhesive dressing is applied directly to the transducer without acoustic coupling gel. Sterile gel is used between the covered probe and the skin. Not all sterile adhesive dressings have favorable acoustic properties for this purpose.

The subclavian artery and the transverse cervical artery are the primary vascular puncture risks of this procedure. Transverse cervical arteries are frequently observed running over or through the brachial plexus in the neck.[9]

Clinical Pearls

- The needle tip should be positioned between the ventral rami of C5, C6, and C7 to ensure complete plexus anesthesia with a multiple-injection technique.[10]
- Arteries that traverse the interscalene brachial plexus can divide it into separate compartments.[11] Multiple injections may be necessary to obtain complete plexus anesthesia when this anatomy is observed.
- The deep cervical artery (the dorsal scapular artery) usually runs between the seventh and eighth cervical roots.[12] This artery continues between the middle and the lower trunks of the brachial plexus.[13]
- The seventh cervical ventral ramus is usually the largest, with progressively smaller cephalad and caudad ventral rami. These size differences tend to equalize the size of the three trunks that form the brachial plexus.

References

1. La Grange P, Foster PA, Pretorius LK. Application of the Doppler ultrasound bloodflow detector in supraclavicular brachial plexus block. *Br J Anaesth.* 1978;50:965-967.
2. Kessler J, Gray AT. Sonography of scalene muscle anomalies for brachial plexus block. *Reg Anesth Pain Med.* 2007;32:172-173.
3. Tubbs RS, Louis RG Jr, Wartmann CT, et al. Histopathological basis for neurogenic thoracic outlet syndrome: laboratory investigation. *J Neurosurg Spine.* 2008;8:347-351.
4. Mangrulkar VH, Cohen HL, Dougherty D. Sonography for diagnosis of cervical ribs in children. *J Ultrasound Med.* 2008;27:1083-1086.
5. Sinha SK, Abrams JH, Weller RS. Ultrasound-guided interscalene needle placement produces successful anesthesia regardless of motor stimulation above or below 0.5 mA. *Anesth Analg.* 2007;105:848-852.
6. Kapral S, Greher M, Huber G, et al. Ultrasonographic guidance improves the success rate of interscalene brachial plexus blockade. *Reg Anesth Pain Med.* 2008;33:253-258.
7. Kessler J, Gray AT. Course of the spinal accessory nerve relative to the brachial plexus. *Reg Anesth Pain Med.* 2007;32:174-176.
8. Tsui BC, Twomey C, Finucane BT. Visualization of the brachial plexus in the supraclavicular region using a curved ultrasound probe with a sterile transparent dressing. *Reg Anesth Pain Med.* 2006;31:182-184.
9. Weiglein AH, Moriggl B, Schalk C, et al. Arteries in the posterior cervical triangle in man. *Clin Anat.* 2005;18:553-557.
10. Koff MD, Cohen JA, McIntyre JJ, et al. Severe brachial plexopathy after an ultrasound-guided single-injection nerve block for total shoulder arthroplasty in a patient with multiple sclerosis. *Anesthesiology.* 2008;108:325-328.
11. Abrahams MS, Panzer O, Atchabahian A, et al. Case report: limitation of local anesthetic spread during ultrasound-guided interscalene block: description of an anatomic variant with clinical correlation. *Reg Anesth Pain Med.* 2008;33:357-359.
12. Demondion X, Herbinet P, Boutry N, et al. Sonographic mapping of the normal brachial plexus. *AJNR Am J Neuroradiol.* 2003;24:1303-1309.
13. Demondion X, Boutry N, Drizenko A, et al. Thoracic outlet: anatomic correlation with MR imaging. *AJR Am J Roentgenol.* 2000;175:417-422.

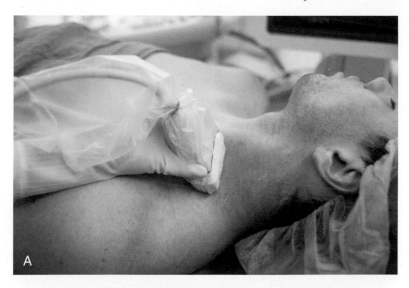

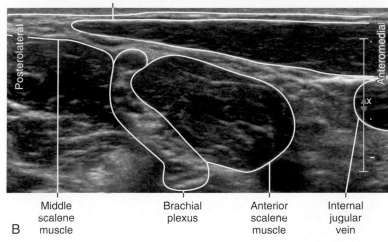

Sternocleidomastoid muscle

Posterolateral

Anteromedial

Middle
scalene
muscle

Brachial
plexus

Anterior
scalene
muscle

Internal
jugular
vein

B

Figure 28-1. External photograph showing the transducer position for interscalene imaging (**A**) and corresponding sonogram (**B**). In this location, the components of the brachial plexus are stacked between the anterior and middle scalene muscles underneath the tapering anterolateral edge of the sternocleidomastoid muscle.

Brachial
plexus

Subclavian
artery

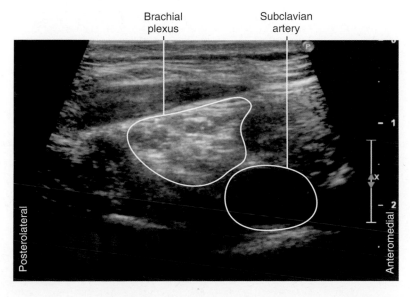

Posterolateral

Anteromedial

Figure 28-2. Supraclavicular imaging. If the probe is moved toward the clavicle and angled caudally, the brachial plexus is seen to bundle compactly in the superior and lateral position with respect to the subclavian artery.

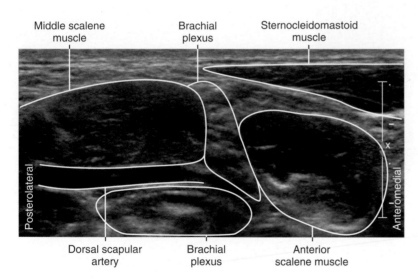

Middle scalene muscle

Brachial plexus

Sternocleidomastoid muscle

Posterolateral

Anteromedial

Dorsal scapular artery

Brachial plexus

Anterior scalene muscle

Figure 28-3. Interscalene imaging reveals a large artery passing through the middle scalene muscle in this subject. The deep cervical artery (the dorsal scapular artery) usually runs between the seventh and eighth cervical roots and can sometimes be identified dividing the middle and the lower trunks of the brachial plexus.

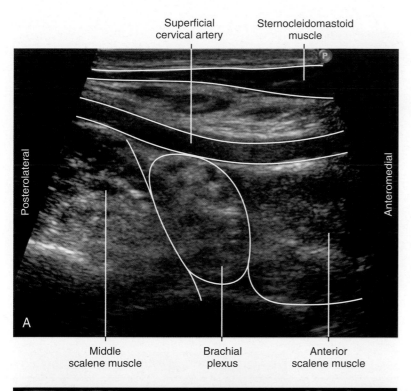

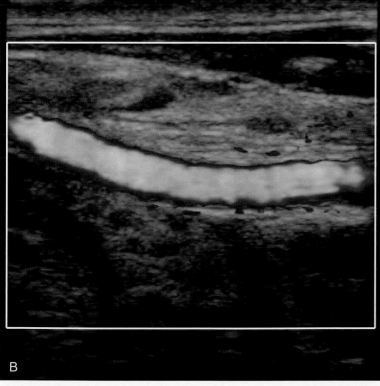

Figure 28-4. B-mode sonogram (**A**) and duplex power Doppler (**B**) identify a superficial cervical artery. The interscalene region is highly vascular. When these vessels are identified, the probe position for interscalene block is moved slightly cephalad or caudad.

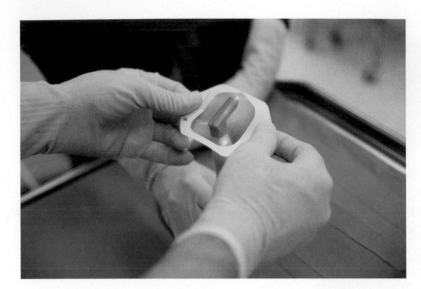

Figure 28-5. Probe cover for interscalene block. A sterile adhesive dressing can be applied to the active face of the transducer and handle. This facilitates needle line-ups with small-footprint transducers.

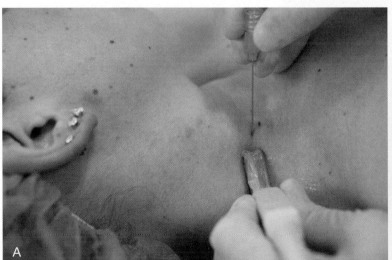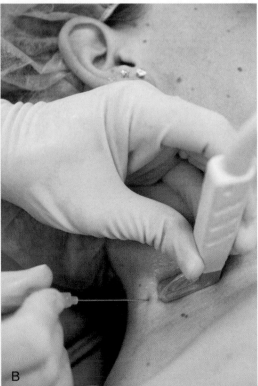

Figure 28-6. External photographs showing in-plane approaches to interscalene block. The medial to lateral approach (**A**) and the lateral to medial approach (**B**) are shown.

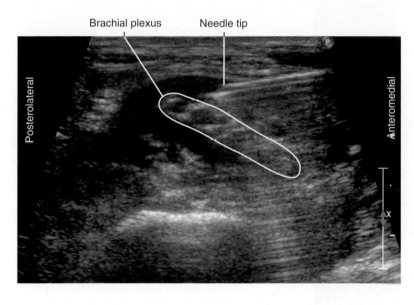

Figure 28-7. Short-axis view of the interscalene plexus during medial to lateral in-plane approach. Local anesthetic is seen to distribute around nerves of the brachial plexus

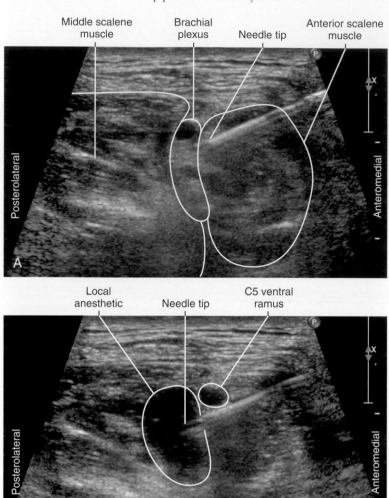

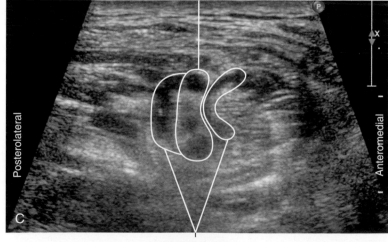

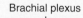

Figure 28-8. Image sequence showing interscalene block. A medial to lateral in-plane approach is demonstrated where the needle tip is carefully placed between components of the plexus (**A** and **B**). After injection, local anesthetic is distributed around both sides of the brachial plexus (**C**).

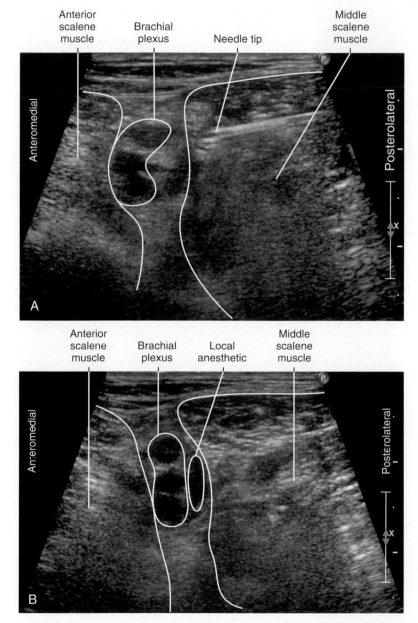

Figure 28-9. Image sequence showing interscalene block. A lateral to medial in-plane approach is demonstrated (**A**). After injection, local anesthetic is distributed around both sides of the brachial plexus (**B**).

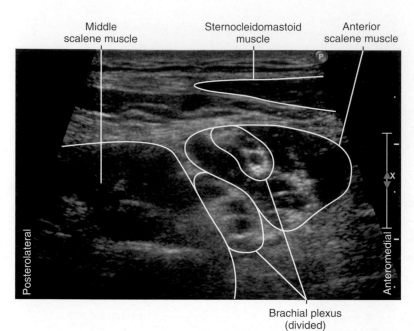

Middle
scalene muscle

Sternocleidomastoid
muscle

Anterior
scalene muscle

Posterolateral

Anteromedial

x

Brachial plexus
(divided)

Figure 28-10. Pass-through brachial plexus. In this sonogram, cephalad elements of the brachial plexus are seen to pass through the anterior scalene muscle. This anatomic variation potentially divides the brachial plexus, with the potential for incomplete blocks.

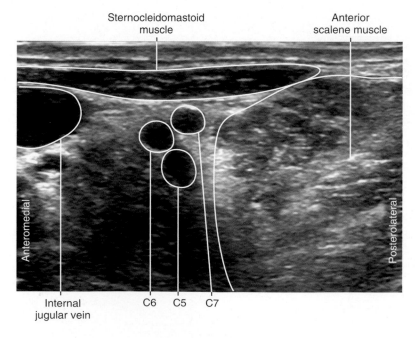

Sternocleidomastoid
muscle

Anterior
scalene muscle

Anteromedial

Posterolateral

Internal
jugular vein

C6   C5   C7

Figure 28-11. Pass-over brachial plexus. In this sonogram, three ventral rami (C5, C6, and C7) are seen to pass over the anterior scalene muscle. It is uncommon for three ventral rami to pass over the anterior scalene, although more commonly, C5 or both C5 and C6 can travel in this pathway.

CHAPTER 29

PHRENIC NERVE IMAGING

The phrenic nerve is a small (<1 mm in diameter), monofascicular nerve that arises from the third, fourth, and fifth cervical ventral rami. The most consistent contribution is from the fourth cervical ventral ramus. At the level of the cricoid cartilage, the phrenic nerve is essentially coincident with the C5 ventral ramus.[1] As the nerve descends the neck, it travels from lateral to medial over the surface of the anterior scalene muscle. The nerve usually enters the chest between the subclavian artery and vein. Accessory phrenic nerves are observed in 60% of specimens and often derive from the fifth cervical ventral ramus.[2]

Phrenic nerve imaging is important for two reasons. First, it may be possible to reduce the incidence of transient pulmonary complications related to phrenic nerve block using ultrasound. Low volumes of local anesthetic (5 mL) administered for interscalene block using ultrasound guidance appear to reduce the incidence of concomitant phrenic nerve block.[3] Ultrasound guidance allows more caudal approaches to brachial plexus block with an even lower chance of phrenic nerve block. Second, direct trauma to the nerve can potentially be avoided during regional anesthetic procedures in the cervical region.

References

1. Kessler J, Schafhalter-Zoppoth I, Gray AT. An ultrasound study of the phrenic nerve in the posterior cervical triangle: implications for the interscalene brachial plexus block. *Reg Anesth Pain Med.* 2008;33:545-550.
2. Loukas M, Kinsella CR Jr, Louis RG Jr, et al. Surgical anatomy of the accessory phrenic nerve. *Ann Thorac Surg.* 2006; 82:1870-1875.
3. Riazi S, Carmichael N, Awad I, et al. Effect of local anaesthetic volume (20 vs 5 mL) on the efficacy and respiratory consequences of ultrasound-guided interscalene brachial plexus block. *Br J Anaesth.* 2008;101:549-556.

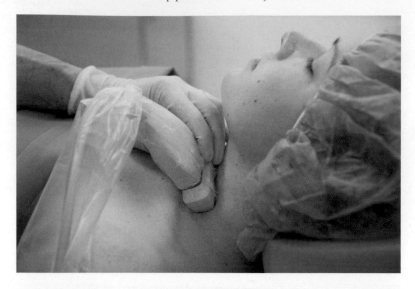

Figure 29-1. External photograph showing the approximate transducer position for phrenic nerve imaging in the cervical region.

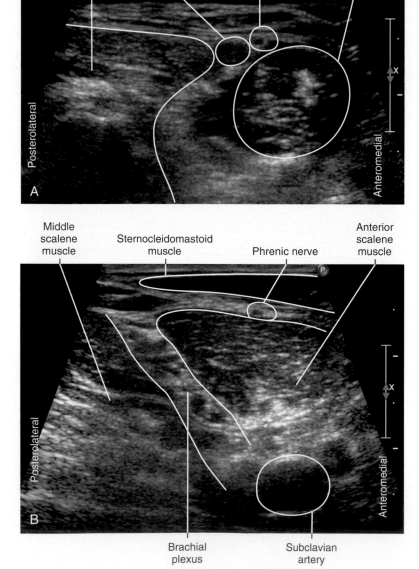

Figure 29-2. Phrenic nerve imaging with ultrasound. At the level of the cricoid cartilage, the phrenic nerve and C5 ventral ramus lie side by side (**A**). At more caudal positions in the neck, the phrenic nerve crosses medially over the surface of the anterior scalene muscle and is visible as monofascicular (**B**).

CHAPTER 30

DORSAL SCAPULAR NERVE IMAGING

The dorsal scapular nerve (DSN) arises from the C5 ventral ramus and frequently contains contributions from C4.[1] The nerve is usually considered part of the brachial plexus. The DSN pierces the middle scalene muscle to innervate the rhomboid muscles and also supplies some of the motor branches to the levator scapulae. The nerve joins the dorsal scapular artery that usually arises from the transverse cervical artery. There is no cutaneous innervation of the DSN.

It is important to recognize the DSN during interscalene blocks of the brachial plexus to avoid trauma to the nerve. The nerve can often be visualized within the middle scalene muscle lateral to the brachial plexus.

Clinical Pearls

- The DSN rounds in shape as it exits the middle scalene muscle, whereas it is flat within this muscle.
- The dorsal scapular artery joins the DSN.

Reference

1. Tubbs RS, Tyler-Kabara EC, Aikens AC, et al. Surgical anatomy of the dorsal scapular nerve. *J Neurosurg.* 2005;102:910-911.

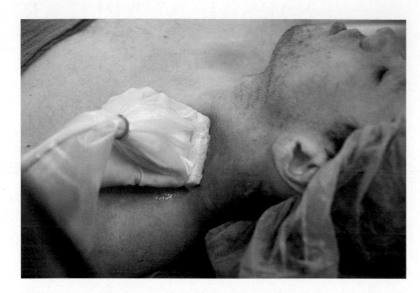

Figure 30-1. External photograph showing the transducer position for imaging the dorsal scapular nerve.

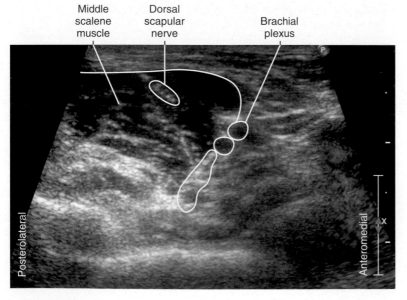

Middle
scalene
muscle

Dorsal
scapular
nerve

Brachial
plexus

Posterolateral

Anteromedial

Figure 30-2. Short-axis view of the dorsal scapular nerve as it leaves the brachial plexus to travel through the middle scalene muscle.

CHAPTER 31

SUPRASCAPULAR NERVE BLOCK

The suprascapular nerve arises from the superior trunk of the brachial plexus, containing contributions from the C5 and C6 ventral rami. The nerve innervates the supraspinatus and infraspinatus muscles and contains articular branches from the shoulder joint. Cutaneous innervation of the suprascapular nerve is not common, being demonstrated in about 15% of subjects.[1,2] When present, the cutaneous distribution is similar to the usual distribution for the axillary nerve.

The suprascapular nerve is about 2 to 3 mm in diameter.[3] The suprascapular nerve diverges distally 2 cm from the junction of C5 and C6 into the superior trunk (range, 0-2.5 cm). The distance measured from the origin of the suprascapular nerve to the clavicle is variable (range, 0.5-7.5 cm).[4] Recognition of the takeoff of the suprascapular nerve from the brachial plexus is important for complete brachial plexus blocks when performed low in the neck. Suprascapular nerve blocks can provide some analgesia after shoulder surgery, but this effect is small.[5] More distal block of the suprascapular nerve near the spinoglenoid notch is potentially more selective, but the nerve and needle imaging for this procedure can be challenging.

Clinical Pearls

- The suprascapular nerve is responsible for most of the sensory innervation to the shoulder joint.[6,7]
- The suprascapular nerve runs parallel to and under the inferior belly of the omohyoid muscle in the posterior triangle of the neck.[8] The suprascapular nerve is accompanied by the suprascapular artery along this course.

References

1. Ajmani ML. The cutaneous branch of the human suprascapular nerve. *J Anat*. 1994;185:439-442.
2. Yan J, Wu H, Aizawa Y, Horiguchi M. The human suprascapular nerve belongs to both anterior and posterior divisions of the brachial plexus. *Okajimas Folia Anat Jpn*. 1999;76:149-155.
3. Aktekin M, Demiryurek D, Bayramoglu A, Tuccar E. The significance of the neurovascular structures passing through the spinoglenoid notch. *Saudi Med J*. 2003;24:933-935.
4. Norkus T, Norkus M, Ramanauskas T. Donor, recipient and nerve grafts in brachial plexus reconstruction: anatomical and technical features for facilitating the exposure. *Surg Radiol Anat*. 2005;27:524-530.
5. Neal JM, McDonald SB, Larkin KL, Polissar NL. Suprascapular nerve block prolongs analgesia after nonarthroscopic shoulder surgery but does not improve outcome. *Anesth Analg*. 2003;96:982-986.
6. Vorster W, Lange CP, Briët RJ, et al. The sensory branch distribution of the suprascapular nerve: an anatomic study. *J Shoulder Elbow Surg*. 2008;17:500-502.
7. Horiguchi M. The cutaneous branch of some human suprascapular nerves. *J Anat*. 1980;130:191-195.
8. Krishnan KG, Pinzer T, Reber F, Schackert G. Endoscopic exploration of the brachial plexus: technique and topographic anatomy. A study in fresh human cadavers. *Neurosurgery*. 2004;54:401-408.

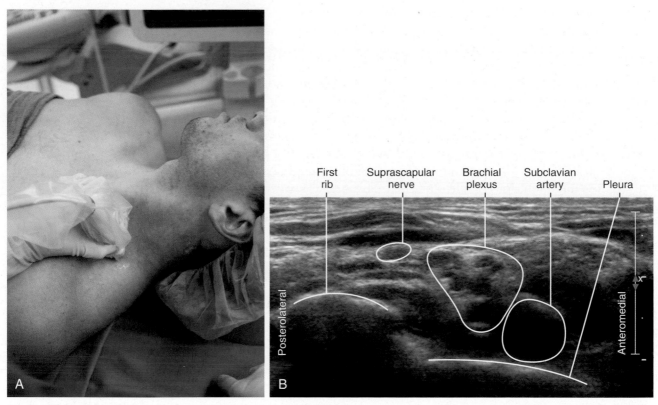

Figure 31-1. External photograph showing the probe position for suprascapular nerve imaging at its takeoff from the brachial plexus (**A**). The corresponding sonogram is also shown (**B**). The suprascapular nerve is responsible for most of the sensory innervation to the shoulder joint.

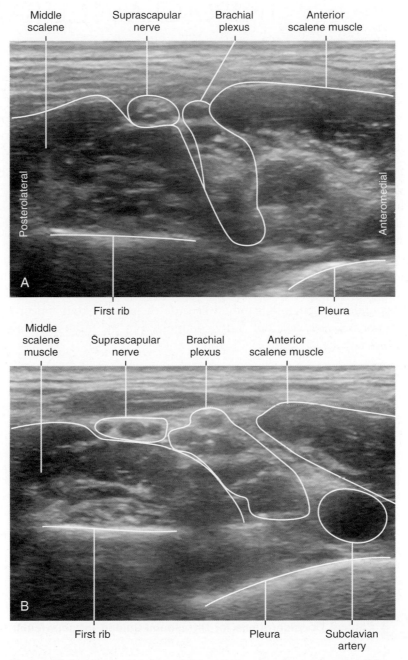

Figure 31-2.   Short-axis views of the suprascapular nerve at the takeoff from the brachial plexus. The nerve diverges superior and lateral to the brachial plexus (**A** and **B**).

CHAPTER 32

INFRACLAVICULAR BLOCK

Infraclavicular block of the brachial plexus was developed because the brachial plexus is relatively compact in this location.[1] For this block, the second part of the axillary artery and the surrounding cords of the brachial plexus are imaged. Because proximal arm muscles are anesthetized (including the pectoralis and deltoid), infraclavicular blocks produce excellent conditions for upper extremity surgery.

The three cords of the brachial plexus (medial, lateral, and posterior) are closely adherent to the second part of the axillary artery beneath the pectoralis minor muscle.[2] The subscapularis muscle separates the infraclavicular brachial plexus from the lung, with a larger margin of safety laterally than medially. The pectoral nerves are sometimes visualized between the pectoralis major and pectoralis minor muscles.

The axillary vein lies on the medial side of the axillary artery, and sometimes the cephalic vein is observed on the lateral side. Otherwise, there are few veins to contend with during the procedure. The cephalic vein passes over the pectoralis minor, whereas the neurovascular bundle passes under the pectoralis minor. Because the axillary vein is deep to the pectoralis major and minor muscles, it is not easily compressed in the infraclavicular space (near the "noncollapsible" subclavian vein).

Suggested Technique

One advantage of infraclavicular block is that the brachial plexus is relatively compact, consisting of three cords. The second part of the axillary artery, which lies under the pectoralis minor muscle, is an excellent landmark for the cords of the brachial plexus. Anatomic variation in this region is uncommon (Table 32-1). Catheters are stable in this location. The block can be performed with the arm abducted or at the side of the patient.

TABLE 32-1	Clinical Considerations for Ultrasound-Guided Infraclavicular Block	
ADVANTAGES		**DISADVANTAGES**
Compact brachial plexus		Deeper block
Anatomic variation uncommon		Specialized equipment (small curved probe)
Stable location for catheters		
Arm positioning		

The major disadvantage of infraclavicular blocks is that the plexus is deep, being covered by both the pectoralis major and pectoralis minor muscles. Therefore, low-frequency, small, curved transducers are favored. Although the block can be performed with the arm at the side, it is still best to abduct the arm if possible to straighten the neurovascular bundle.[3] Because the block is deep, a large-bore needle is recommended (17 or 18 gauge) to improve needle tip visibility.[4]

The fascial layers under the pectoralis minor and over the subscapularis are effective for containing local anesthetic. The injections should ideally separate the cords from the artery by placing the needle tip between each of the three cords and the artery. If a catheter is placed, the posterior position appears to result in the most consistent brachial plexus anesthesia.

Clinical Pearls

- For ultrasound-guided infraclavicular block, the sensory block rate of the axillary nerve is in the 60% to 80% range.[3]
- Pectoral nerves can often be identified between the pectoralis major and pectoralis minor muscles.[5-7]
- When the upper arm is abducted 90 degrees, the brachial plexus is closer to the skin and farther from the pleura compared with other positions.[8,9]

References

1. Raj PP, Montgomery SJ, Nettles D, Jenkins MT. Infraclavicular brachial plexus block: a new approach. *Anesth Analg.* 1973; 52:897-904.
2. Sauter AR, Smith HJ, Stubhaug A, et al. Use of magnetic resonance imaging to define the anatomical location closest to all three cords of the infraclavicular brachial plexus. *Anesth Analg.* 2006;103:1574-1576.
3. Bigeleisen P, Wilson M. A comparison of two techniques for ultrasound guided infraclavicular block. *Br J Anaesth.* 2006; 96:502-507.
4. Sandhu NS, Manne JS, Medabalmi PK, Capan LM. Sonographically guided infraclavicular brachial plexus block in adults: a retrospective analysis of 1146 cases. *J Ultrasound Med.* 2006;25:1555-1561.
5. Macchi V, Tiengo C, Porzionato A, et al. Medial and lateral pectoral nerves: course and branches. *Clin Anat.* 2007;20:157-162.
6. Aszmann OC, Rab M, Kamolz L, Frey M. The anatomy of the pectoral nerves and their significance in brachial plexus reconstruction. *J Hand Surg [Am].* 2000;25:942-947.
7. Hoffman GW, Elliott LF. The anatomy of the pectoral nerves and its significance to the general and plastic surgeon. *Ann Surg.* 1987;205:504-507.
8. Wang FY, Wu SH, Lu IC, et al. Ultrasonographic examination to search out the optimal upper arm position for coracoid approach to infraclavicular brachial plexus block: a volunteer study. *Acta Anaesthesiol Taiwan.* 2007;45:15-20.
9. Unlu E, Sen T, Esmer AF, et al. A new technique for subscapularis muscle needle insertion. *Am J Phys Med Rehabil.* 2008;87:710-713.

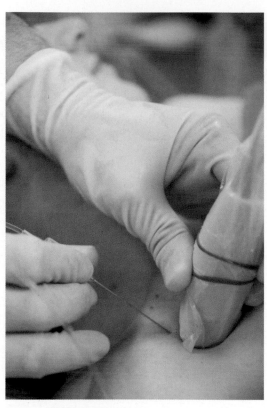

Figure 32-1. External photograph showing the approach to infraclavicular block. An in-plane approach from the head of the table is shown. A curved probe is chosen because of the working room limitation imposed by the clavicle. If possible, the arm should be abducted to straighten the neurovascular bundle for infraclavicular block.

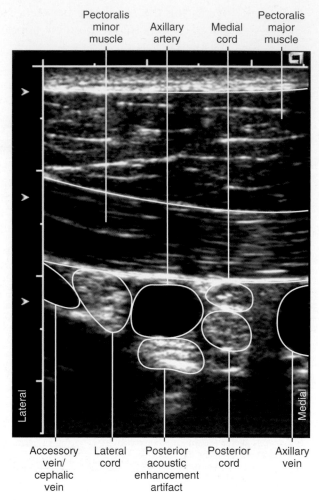

Figure 32-2. Short-axis view of the second part of the axillary artery under the pectoralis major and pectoralis minor muscles. The cords of the brachial plexus are named for their position with respect to the artery. The three cords of the brachial plexus have a triangular arrangement around the second part of the axillary artery, which lies underneath the pectoralis minor muscle. The clavipectoral fascia creates a favorable space for injection of local anesthetic and catheter placement in the infraclavicular region.

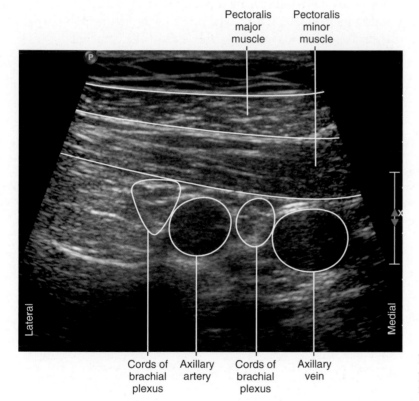

Pectoralis major muscle

Pectoralis minor muscle

Lateral

Medial

Cords of brachial plexus

Axillary artery

Cords of brachial plexus

Axillary vein

Figure 32-3. Sonogram of the infraclavicular brachial plexus displayed in wide-screen format. Most practitioners favor a small-footprint transducer with a broad view.

CHAPTER 33

AXILLARY BLOCK

Three terminal branches of the brachial plexus (the median, radial, and ulnar nerves) lie close to the axillary artery in the axilla (Table 33-1). This makes the axilla a convenient place to block the brachial plexus (Table 33-2). Axillary block is traditionally performed by transarterial injection of local anesthetic around the axillary artery or by use of nerve stimulation to evoke motor responses. Transarterial block necessitates puncturing the axillary artery. Another weakness is failure to anesthetize the musculocutaneous nerve, which leaves the neurovascular bundle proximally underneath the pectoralis minor muscle at the level of the coracoid process.

TABLE 33-1	Characteristics of Terminal Branches of the Brachial Plexus in the Axilla
NERVE	**CHARACTERISTICS**
Axillary	Accompanies posterior circumflex humeral artery Takeoff is proximal to teres major and latissimus dorsi tendons
Musculocutaneous	Lateral course through coracobrachialis Flat shape when inside this muscle If not visible, rule out median-musculocutaneous nerve fusion
Radial	Accompanies profunda brachii artery Travels to spiral groove of humerus Takeoff is distal to teres major and latissimus dorsi tendons
Median	Can be displaced to side of axillary artery with compression Accompanies brachial artery
Ulnar	Lies between axillary artery and vein Acoustic window through axillary vein Most consistent position (at 2- to 3-o'clock position with respect to artery) Travels to cubital tunnel
Medial antebrachial cutaneous	Lies between median nerve and ulnar nerve
Intercostobrachial and medial brachial cutaneous	Lie within the subcutaneous tissue of the medial arm Medial to brachial artery

TABLE 33-2	Clinical Considerations for Axillary Block With Ultrasound	
ADVANTAGES		**DISADVANTAGES**
Shallow nerves		Divergent plexus
Working room		Anatomic variation
Compressible site		Arm positioning
Remote from the lung		Multiple veins
No risk for phrenic nerve block		Catheters problematic

Ultrasound imaging improves axillary block of the brachial plexus. Almost all institutions have reported advantages to using ultrasound to guide this procedure.[1,2] Ultrasound can be used to guide injections around the axillary artery. In addition, the musculocutaneous nerve can be directly imaged for regional block (see Chapter 34).

Suggested Technique

The transpectoral approach for proximal axillary block is performed with the needle tip just inside the chest, before the nerves of the brachial plexus diverge. With this lateral to medial approach, the needle enters through the pectoralis major muscle.

Axillary block is performed with the patient in supine position. The arm should be slightly hyperabducted to allow the needle placement to be as proximal as possible. Slightly more than 90 degrees of abduction is optimal for probe positioning. Because the pectoralis major inserts on the humerus, hyperabduction of the arm will reduce the pectoral ridge by retracting the pectoralis major toward the midline. A Mayo stand can be used to support the arm in this position. The operator should stand at the head of the bed to view the ultrasound display across the patient's arm.

The pectoral ridge will separate the needle entry point and the transducer for this proximal axillary block. This can allow for coverless imaging because the needle entry site is remote from the transducer. The skin preparation is over the pectoralis major muscle. Tilting and rotating the angle of the transducer slightly into the chest torso allows for more proximal imaging. The axillary veins can be used as a manometer to measure the amount of probe compression. The correct amount of pressure for this procedure just coapts the walls of the veins.

Structures potentially in the needle path when approaching the axillary neurovascular bundle are the cephalic vein, the tendon of the pectoralis major, and the musculocutaneous nerve. The cephalic vein lies in the deltopectoral groove; therefore, there is a low potential for venous puncture as the needle enters the skin.

The conjoint tendon of the latissimus dorsi and teres major inserts on the humerus and is a valuable landmark for this procedure. The radial nerve takeoff from the axillary artery is always distal to this tendon. The needle should enter the skin away from the transducer so that it approaches slightly deep to the artery and can easily be placed between the artery and conjoint tendon for injection.

Because the axillary artery and wall-hugging nerves of the brachial plexus (median, radial, and ulnar) are surrounded by common connective tissue, the ideal place for block needle tip placement is between the nerves and the artery. If this is done, the perivascular injections will separate the nerves from the artery. Injections at the outside corner of the nerves (away from the axillary artery) also can be successful, but careful assessment must show that the injection actually encircles the nerves.

Local anesthetic injections are made in front and in back of the axillary artery. The injection in back of the artery is typically done first. This will bring the neurovascular bundle even closer to the skin surface. The musculocutaneous nerve is blocked separately (see Chapter 34).

It is especially important for the front-wall injection to be between the median nerve and the axillary artery. The median nerve crosses the front surface of the axillary artery. If local anesthetic tracks proximally along the median nerve to its medial and lateral cord contributions, two thirds of the brachial plexus will be anesthetized. The median, ulnar, medial antebrachial cutaneous, and musculocutaneous nerves derive from the medial and lateral cords.

The intercostobrachial nerves (from T1 and T2) are not part of the brachial plexus but contribute to sensory innervation of the medial arm. Intercostobrachial nerve block can be achieved by subcutaneous infiltration of the medial arm at the axillary crease. Imaging guidance is not necessary for this procedure.

Clinical Pearls

- With this proximal approach to axillary block, the needle will naturally be channeled into the space between the axillary artery and conjoint tendon of the latissimus dorsi and teres major for the posterior injection. A slight upward trajectory is all that is needed to steer the needle along and above this tendon complex.
- With classic approaches to axillary block, the radial nerve is often spared.[3]

References

1. Soeding PE, Sha S, Royse CE, et al. A randomized trial of ultrasound-guided brachial plexus anaesthesia in upper limb surgery. *Anaesth Intensive Care.* 2005;33:719-725.
2. Lo N, Brull R, Perlas A, et al. Evolution of ultrasound guided axillary brachial plexus blockade: retrospective analysis of 662 blocks. *Can J Anaesth.* 2008;55:408-413.
3. Lanz E, Theiss D, Jankovic D. The extent of blockade following various techniques of brachial plexus block. *Anesth Analg.* 1983;62:55-58.

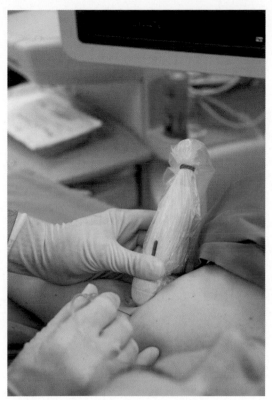

Figure 33-1. External photograph showing the approach to axillary block. An in-plane approach from the lateral aspect of the arm is shown. Slight reverse Trendelenburg position (or elevation of the head of the bed) will make the needle path more natural for the operator. The display is placed across the arm board (not across the operating table).

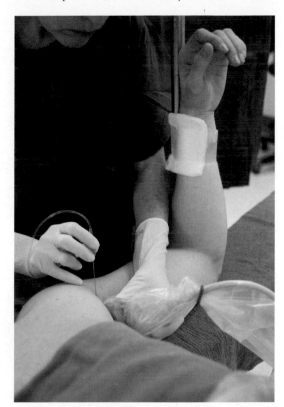

Figure 33-2. Arm position for axillary block, chosen based on range of motion of the arm. When there is some limitation of motion, the arm can be taped to an intravenous pole for stabilization. With severe limitation of motion, the arm can be placed near the side with just enough room to place the transducer in the axilla. Contrary to popular belief, less range of motion is necessary for ultrasound-guided axillary block than with traditional approaches.

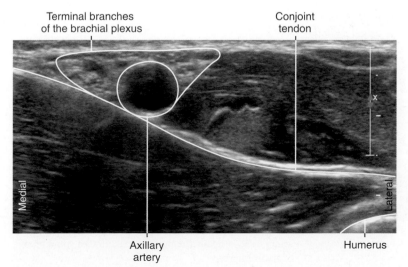

Figure 33-3. Short-axis view of the axillary artery and surrounding branches of the brachial plexus in the axilla. The conjoint tendon of the teres major and latissimus dorsi lies under the neurovascular bundle. Because the radial nerve takeoff is distal to the conjoint tendon, visualization of this structure ensures a compact brachial plexus suitable for complete block.

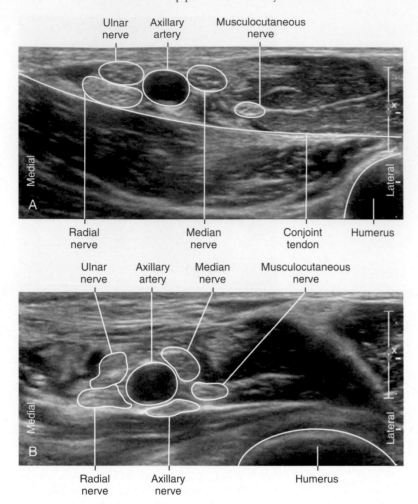

Figure 33-4. Short-axis views of the brachial plexus from probe manipulation in the axilla. With some subjects, the axillary nerve can be viewed posterior to the axillary artery by tilting the probe into the chest. Both distal (**A**) and proximal (**B**) views are shown.

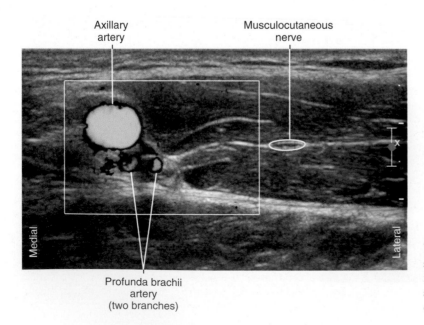

Figure 33-5. The profunda brachii artery shown in short-axis view with power Doppler imaging. The profunda brachii artery exits the back wall of the axillary artery to accompany the radial nerve into the spiral groove of the humerus.

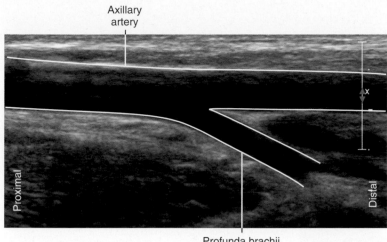

Axillary
artery

Proximal

Distal

Profunda brachii
artery

Figure 33-6. The profunda brachii artery shown in long-axis view with B-mode imaging.

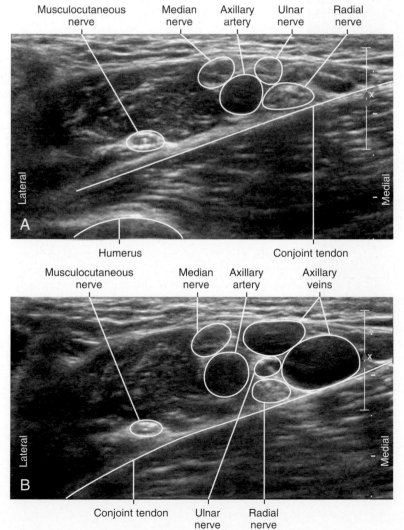

Musculocutaneous
nerve

Median
nerve

Axillary
artery

Ulnar
nerve

Radial
nerve

Lateral

Medial

A

Humerus

Conjoint tendon

Musculocutaneous
nerve

Median
nerve

Axillary
artery

Axillary
veins

Lateral

Medial

B

Conjoint tendon

Ulnar
nerve

Radial
nerve

Figure 33-7. Axillary scout view imaging to look for veins before needle placement. Images are shown with (**A**) and without (**B**) probe compression. During needle placement, the vein walls are maintained coapted to reduce the chance of venous puncture.

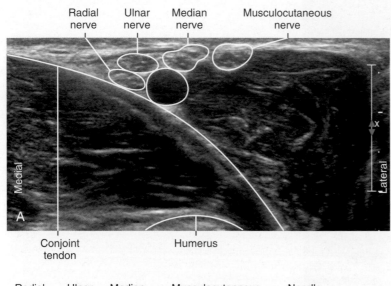

Radial nerve   Ulnar nerve   Median nerve   Musculocutaneous nerve

Medial

Lateral

x

A

Conjoint tendon   Humerus

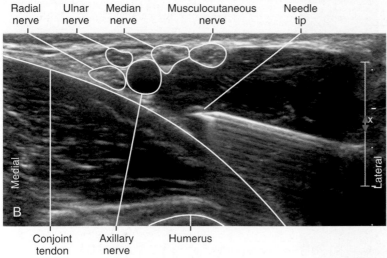

Radial nerve   Ulnar nerve   Median nerve   Musculocutaneous nerve   Needle tip

Medial

Lateral

x

B

Conjoint tendon   Axillary nerve   Humerus

Figure 33-8. In-plane approach to axillary block. Sonograms are shown before (**A**) and after (**B**) needle placement. With this approach, the needle will naturally be channeled into the space between the axillary artery and conjoint tendon of the latissimus dorsi and teres major for the posterior injection. A slight upward trajectory is all that is needed to steer the needle along and above the tendon complex.

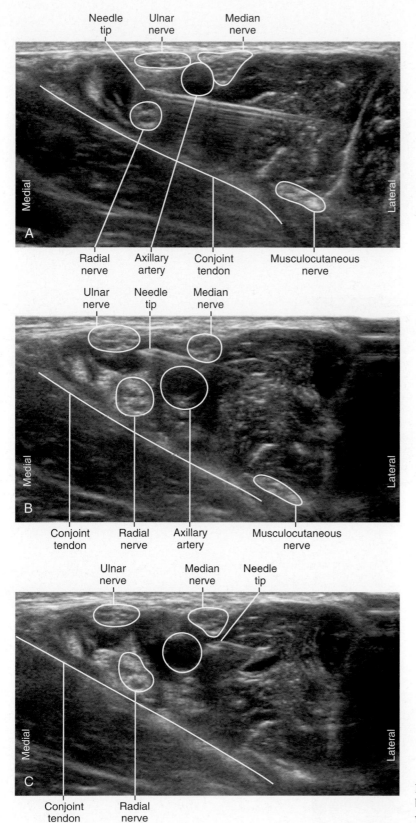

Figure 33-9. Axillary block image sequence showing back-wall injection (**A**), front-wall injection (**B**), and front-wall injection as the needle is removed (**C**).

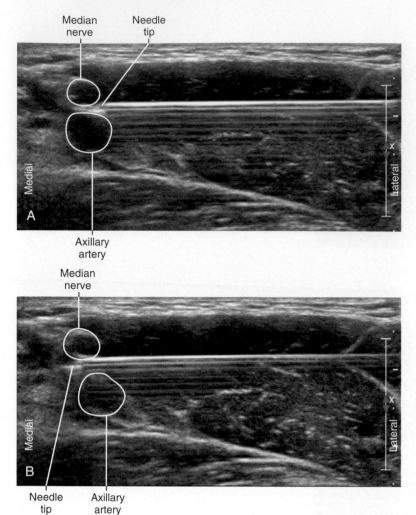

Median nerve   Needle tip

Medial

Lateral

A

Axillary artery

Median nerve

Medial

Lateral

B

Needle tip   Axillary artery

Figure 33-10. Axillary block image sequence. The block needle approaches the gap between the median nerve and axillary artery (**A**). As the needle is advanced and local anesthetic is slowly injected, the nerve and artery are separated (**B**). The beveled needle can be used as a shovel to scoop up the peripheral nerve and carry it away from adjacent structures (e.g., arteries or other peripheral nerves).

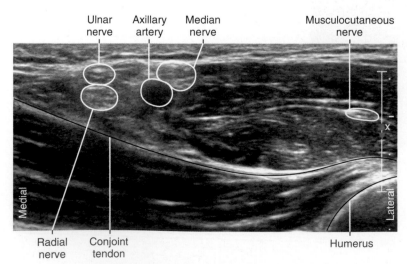

Ulnar nerve   Axillary artery   Median nerve   Musculocutaneous nerve

Medial

Lateral

Radial nerve   Conjoint tendon   Humerus

Figure 33-11. Short-axis view of the axillary artery after axillary block. After successful injection, the local anesthetic separates the nerves from the axillary artery.

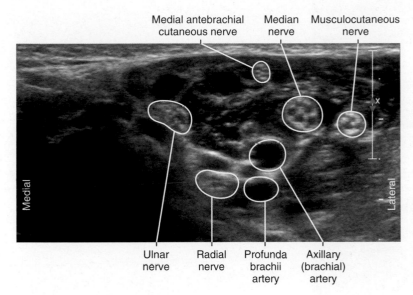

Medial antebrachial cutaneous nerve

Median nerve

Musculocutaneous nerve

Medial

Lateral

Ulnar nerve

Radial nerve

Profunda brachii artery

Axillary (brachial) artery

Figure 33-12. Short-axis view of the medial antebrachial cutaneous nerve after axillary block. After injection, this small nerve can often be identified between the median and ulnar nerves toward the skin surface. Visible separation of the wall-hugging nerves from the axillary artery ensures successful axillary block.

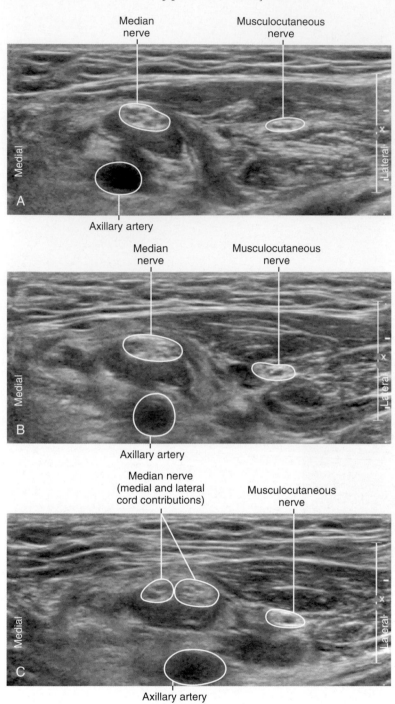

Figure 33-13. Median nerve after axillary block in short-axis view from distal (**A**) and proximal (**B** and **C**). The median nerve derives from both the medal and lateral cord, and these contributions can often be identified after successful axillary block because the local anesthetic tracks proximally to provide reverse acoustic contrast.

Axillary
artery

Median
nerve

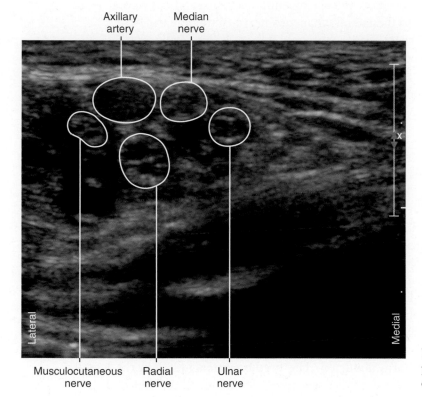

Lateral

Medial

x

Musculocutaneous
nerve

Radial
nerve

Ulnar
nerve

Figure 33-14. Short-axis view after axillary block in a young child. The axillary block is a versatile block applicable in many clinical circumstances.

CHAPTER 34

MUSCULOCUTANEOUS NERVE BLOCK

The musculocutaneous nerve is a branch of the lateral cord of the brachial plexus. The nerve innervates the flexors of the arm at the elbow (biceps brachii, brachialis, and coracobrachialis muscles). The nerve also gives rise to the lateral cutaneous nerve of the forearm.

The musculocutaneous nerve usually passes through the coracobrachialis muscle. The musculocutaneous nerve exits the coracobrachialis between its two parts and the short head of the biceps, forming a triangle with these three muscular components. The musculocutaneous nerve will lie between the biceps and the brachialis more distally.

Suggested Technique

Ultrasound imaging of the musculocutaneous nerve in the axilla can be used to facilitate regional block.[1] This directly addresses one of the primary weaknesses of traditional axillary block.

The lateral course of the nerve and its changes in shape as it passes through the coracobrachialis muscle are characteristic features that allow ultrasound identification of the nerve.[2] The nerve is typically flat within the coracobrachialis muscle; therefore, this is a desirable location for regional block. The relatively high surface area–to-volume ratio may improve onset kinetics of the block.

The block is performed with the arm abducted. The needle approaches from the lateral side of the arm. The choices of transducer and block needle are not critical. The needle tip is positioned at the lateral corner of the musculocutaneous nerve within the fascial plane of the coracobrachialis muscle that contains the nerve in the axilla.

The lateral cutaneous branch of the musculocutaneous nerve can be more selectively blocked distal to the nerve exit from the coracobrachialis muscle. The point of exit is usually easy to identify because the nerve has a triangular shape in that location.[2] Blockade of the more proximal motor fibers of the musculocutaneous nerve is unlikely with this approach. However, the nerve to the biceps brachii continues for about 4 cm after the exit from the coracobrachialis before branching off.[3]

The estimated incidence of pass-over musculocutaneous nerve (musculocutaneous nerve path over the coracobrachialis muscle rather than through it) ranges from 8% to 30%.[4-6] This usually does not present a problem because the nerve can be directly imaged.

Fusion of the median nerve and musculocutaneous nerve is another common anomaly (a low-lying lateral cord). In these fusion products, the median contribution is typically larger and more superficial than the musculocutaneous contribution.[7] Small muscular branches can sometimes be identified that course medial to lateral from the musculocutaneous contribution.

In some patients, the lateral cutaneous nerve of the forearm extends to the dorsal aspect of the thumb (musculocutaneous dominance of the dorsum of the hand). Local anesthetic infiltration through the anatomic snuffbox will block both superficial radial and musculocutaneous contributions to the dorsum of the hand.

References

1. Spence BC, Sites BD, Beach ML. Ultrasound-guided musculocutaneous nerve block: a description of a novel technique. *Reg Anesth Pain Med.* 2005;30:198-201.
2. Schafhalter-Zoppoth I, Gray AT. The musculocutaneous nerve: ultrasound appearance for peripheral nerve block. *Reg Anesth Pain Med.* 2005;30:385-390.
3. Macchi V, Tiengo C, Porzionato A, et al. Musculocutaneous nerve: histotopographic study and clinical implications. *Clin Anat.* 2007;20:400-406.
4. Flatow EL, Bigliani LU, April EW. An anatomic study of the musculocutaneous nerve and its relationship to the coracoid process. *Clin Orthop.* 1989;244:166-171.
5. el-Naggar MM. A study on the morphology of the coracobrachialis muscle and its relationship with the musculocutaneous nerve. *Folia Morphol (Warsz).* 2001;60:217-224.
6. Eglseder WA Jr, Goldman M. Anatomic variations of the musculocutaneous nerve in the arm. *Am J Orthop.* 1997;26:777-780.
7. Orebaugh SL, Pennington S. Variant location of the musculocutaneous nerve during axillary nerve block. *J Clin Anesth.* 2006;18:541-544.

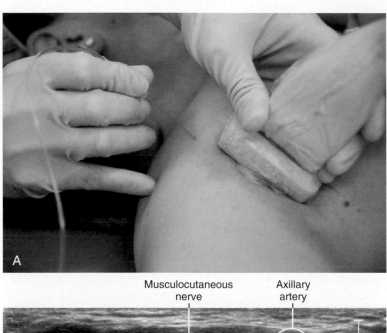

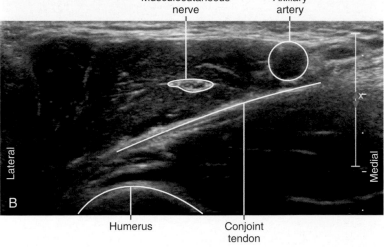

Figure 34-1. External photograph showing the approach to musculocutaneous nerve block in the axilla (**A**). An in-plane approach from the lateral aspect of the forearm is shown. The corresponding sonogram before needle placement is shown (**B**).

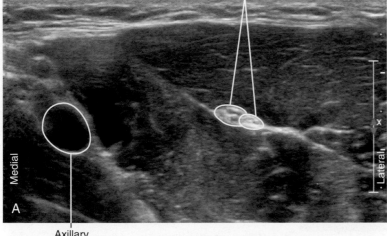

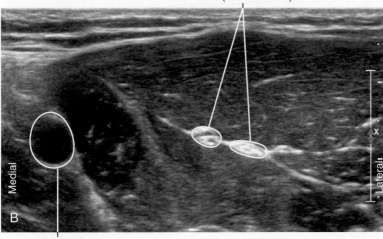

Figure 34-2. Division of the musculocutaneous nerve into anterior and posterior branches in the distal arm. Sonograms are shown proximal (**A**) and distal (**B**) to the division. Musculocutaneous nerve blocks are usually performed proximally for more complete anesthesia.

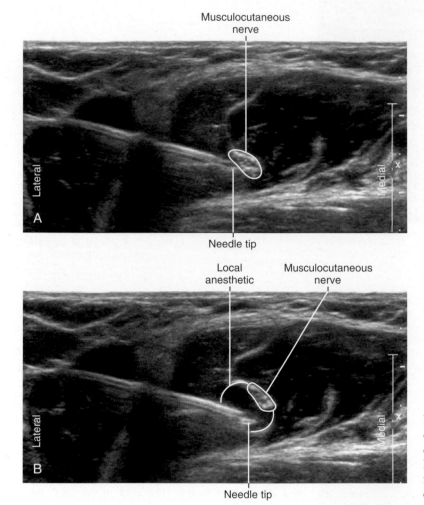

Figure 34-3. Image sequence showing musculocutaneous nerve block in the axilla. An in-plane approach is demonstrated whereby the needle tip is placed under the lateral aspect of the musculocutaneous nerve (A). After injection, local anesthetic is distributed around the musculocutaneous nerve (B).

Musculocutaneous
nerve

Local
anesthetic

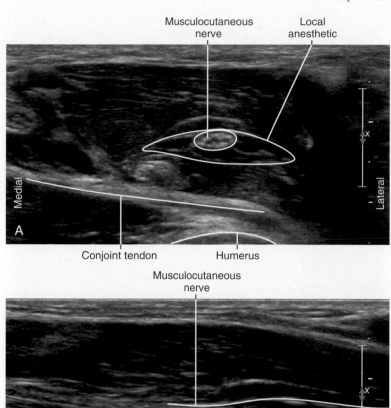

Medial

Lateral

A

Conjoint tendon   Humerus

Musculocutaneous
nerve

Proximal

Distal

B

Local anesthetic

Figure 34-4. Distribution of local anesthetic after musculocutaneous nerve block in the axilla. After injection, local anesthetic is distributed around the musculocutaneous nerve as seen in short-axis view (**A**) and tracks along the nerve as seen in long-axis view (**B**).

Median
nerve

Axillary (brachial)
artery

Ulnar nerve

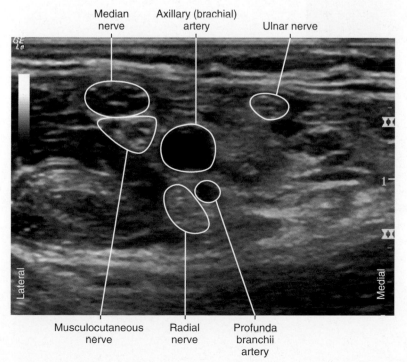

Lateral

Medial

Musculocutaneous
nerve

Radial
nerve

Profunda
branchii
artery

Figure 34-5. Musculocutaneous-median nerve fusion (low-lying lateral cord). In this variation, the two nerves are together in the axilla. Muscular and cutaneous branches may split off directly from the fusion product more distally in the arm.

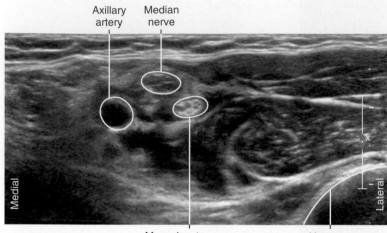

Axillary artery   Median nerve

Medial

Lateral

Musculocutaneous nerve

Humerus

Figure 34-6. Musculocutaneous-median nerve fusion (low-lying lateral cord). After regional block, local anesthetic separates this fusion product.

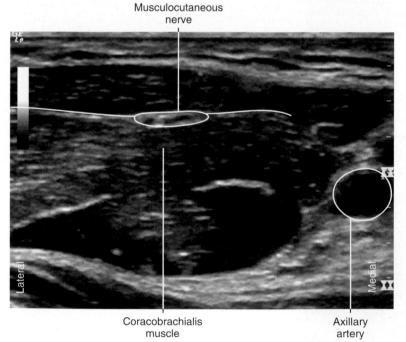

Musculocutaneous nerve

Lateral

Medial

Coracobrachialis muscle

Axillary artery

Figure 34-7. Pass-over musculocutaneous nerve. In most individuals, the musculocutaneous nerve passes through the coracobrachialis muscle. However, in some individuals, the musculocutaneous nerve passes over the muscle. Under most circumstances, the nerve can be directly imaged, thereby facilitating regional block.

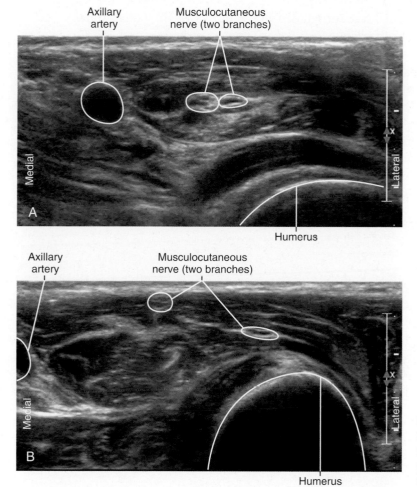

Figure 34-8. In some individuals, a large cutaneous branch of the musculocutaneous nerve can be identified that travels to the skin of the lateral arm (**A** and **B**). When present, this branch may be important for arm tourniquet tolerance.

CHAPTER 35

FOREARM BLOCKS

Peripheral blocks of terminal branches of the brachial plexus (median, radial, and ulnar nerves) can offer benefits in terms of patient disposition.[1,2] These procedures can be used to prevent and treat postoperative pain. Ultrasound-guided nerve blocks of the radial, ulnar, and median nerves are also useful in the emergency department to provide anesthesia for hand procedures.[3]

Forearm blocks provide sensory anesthesia of the hand and block the intrinsic muscles of the hand. However, the extrinsic muscles (the more proximal branches to the flexors and extensors of the digits) are spared, and therefore some hand motion is possible. Forearm blocks are useful for trigger finger release when active motion is desired and other minor surgical procedures of the hand that do not require a tourniquet. Because forearm blocks anesthetize the proximal palmar and dorsal cutaneous nerves of the hand, these blocks are usually more complete than conventional wrist blocks. Because the flexors and extensors of the arm at the elbow are spared, no arm sling is necessary following forearm blocks.

References

1. Gebhard RE, Al-Samsam T, Greger J, et al. Distal nerve blocks at the wrist for outpatient carpal tunnel surgery offer intraoperative cardiovascular stability and reduce discharge time. *Anesth Analg.* 2002;95:351-355.
2. Gray AT, Schafhalter-Zoppoth I. Ultrasound guidance for ulnar nerve block in the forearm. *Reg Anesth Pain Med.* 2003; 28:335-339.
3. Liebmann O, Price D, Mills C, et al. Feasibility of forearm ultrasonography-guided nerve blocks of the radial, ulnar, and median nerves for hand procedures in the emergency department. *Ann Emerg Med.* 2006;48:558-562.

CHAPTER 36

RADIAL NERVE BLOCK

The radial nerve is a branch of the posterior cord of the brachial plexus. It provides motor innervation to the extensor-supinator group of muscles. Of the three nerves that surround the axillary artery in the axilla (median, radial, and ulnar), the radial nerve is the most difficult to visualize and access with the block needle.[1]

The radial nerve has branches all along its course, including the posterior cutaneous branch of the forearm (sensory), deep radial nerve (motor), and superficial radial nerve (sensory).

The posterior cutaneous branch of the forearm diverges from the radial nerve about 16 cm proximal to the lateral epicondyle of the humerus.[2] This branch provides sensation to both the elbow joint and posterior forearm.

The radial nerve divides into its superficial and deep branches in the antecubital fossa over the lateral epicondyle of the humerus. The radial nerve often has a snake-eyes appearance before this separation. The superficial radial nerve is slightly medial to the deep radial nerve within a fascial plane in this location. The deep radial nerve can be easily viewed crossing through the supinator muscle by sliding the transducer back and forth just distal to the lateral epicondyle with the arm pronated. This is a useful starting point to help find the common radial nerve and its superficial branch, which can be more difficult to visualize.

The superficial radial nerve joins the lateral side of the radial artery in the middle third of the forearm. The superficial radial nerve travels the lateral forearm just deep to the brachioradialis muscle. Most patients have radial dominance of sensation of the dorsal aspect of the hand, as primarily supplied by the superficial branch of the radial nerve.[3]

Suggested Technique

The superficial radial nerve can be blocked in the proximal third of the forearm before it joins the lateral side of the radial artery and divides into smaller branches.[4] In this location, the superficial radial nerve is covered by the brachioradialis as it travels over the supinator muscle. An in-plane approach from the lateral side of the forearm works well with the block needle tip placed under the nerve. The arm is pronated to facilitate placement of the needle. Similarly, the radial nerve can be blocked slightly more proximally in the antecubital fossa before the nerve divides into superficial (sensory) and deep (motor) branches.

The radial nerve also can be blocked in the distal arm after the nerve emerges from the spiral groove of the humerus. The radial nerve lies within the fascia that divides the brachioradialis from the underlying brachialis muscle. The arm is pronated and elevated to facilitate imaging of the nerve in the posterolateral arm for the block procedure. The radial nerve is round or oval in this location. The injection targets the fascial plane between the brachialis (deep) and brachioradialis (superficial). The posterior cutaneous nerve of the forearm lies superficial and posterior to the radial nerve above the elbow, so injection on pullback of the needle is advised to ensure complete block.

The radial nerve emerges from the spiral groove where the lateral intermuscular septum inserts on the humerus. This insertion creates the lateral supracondylar ridge along the bone. Because the lateral intermuscular septum separates the brachioradialis from the triceps, the ridge will point behind to the radial nerve. The radial nerve travels anteriorly after emerging from the spiral groove of the humerus. The nerve travels within the fascia between the brachialis and brachioradialis muscles.

Neurologic Assessment

Sensory block of the radial nerve can be tested at the dorsal web between the index finger and thumb. Motor block of the deep radial nerve results in wrist drop.

References

1. Chan VW, Perlas A, McCartney CJ, et al. Ultrasound guidance improves success rate of axillary brachial plexus block. *Can J Anaesth.* 2007;54:176-182.
2. MacAvoy MC, Rust SS, Green DP. Anatomy of the posterior antebrachial cutaneous nerve: practical information for the surgeon operating on the lateral aspect of the elbow. *J Hand Surg [Am].* 2006;31:908-911.
3. Auerbach DM, Collins ED, Kunkle KL, Monsanto EH. The radial sensory nerve. An anatomic study. *Clin Orthop Relat Res.* 1994;(308):241-249.
4. Ikiz ZA, Ucerler H. Anatomic characteristics and clinical importance of the superficial branch of the radial nerve. *Surg Radiol Anat.* 2004;26:453-458.

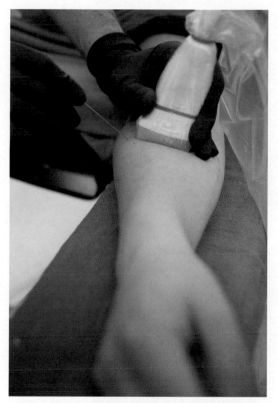

Figure 36-1. External photograph showing the approach to superficial radial nerve block in the proximal forearm. An in-plane approach from the lateral aspect of the forearm is shown.

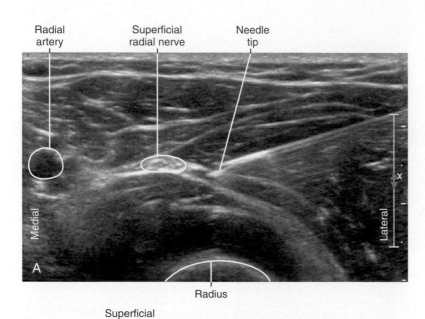

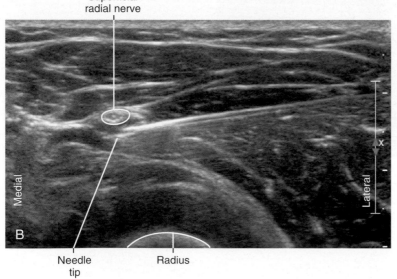

Figure 36-2. Image sequence showing superficial radial nerve block in the forearm. An in-plane approach is demonstrated where the needle tip is placed under the superficial radial nerve (**A**). After injection, local anesthetic is distributed around the superficial radial nerve resulting in sensory block of the dorsum of the hand (**B**).

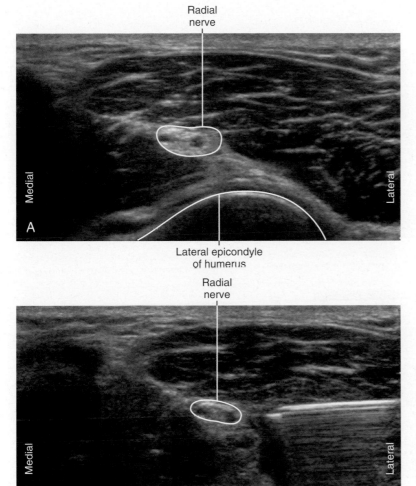

Figure 36-3. Snake-eyes appearance to the radial nerve in the antecubital fossa (**A**). The snake-eyes appearance consists of both the superficial (sensory) and deep (motor) branches before the deep branch dives through the supinator muscle. In-plane approach to radial nerve block from the lateral aspect of the arm (**B**). If the radial nerve is blocked in this location, the motor block will result in wrist drop.

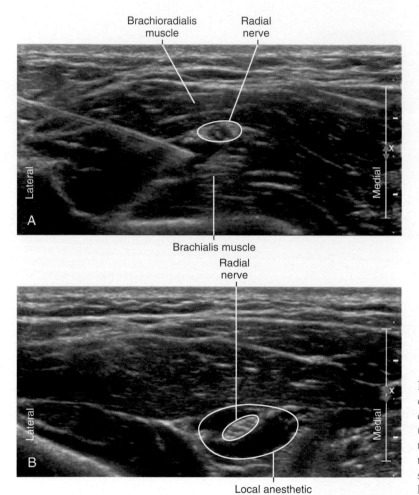

Figure 36-4. Short-axis view of the radial nerve in the distal arm between the spiral groove and the lateral epicondyle of the humerus showing the block needle in place (**A**). The brachialis muscle separates the radial nerve from the underlying bone. The brachioradialis muscle covers the radial nerve. After injection, local anesthetic is seen to surround the radial nerve (**B**). Radial nerve block in this location will result in both sensory and motor block.

CHAPTER 37

MEDIAN NERVE BLOCK

The median nerve is a branch of the medial and lateral cords of the brachial plexus. The median nerve provides most of the sensory innervation to the palm of the hand. It is part of the neurovascular bundle in the axilla and continues with the brachial artery on its medial side proximal to the elbow.

In the forearm, the median nerve lies between the flexor digitorum profundus and the flexor digitorum superficialis muscles. This is where the median nerve is usually brightest on ultrasound scans.[1]

The two largest branches of the median nerve are the anterior interosseous nerve and the palmar cutaneous branch. About 5 to 8 cm distal to the lateral epicondyle, the anterior interosseous nerve (a purely motor nerve) branches off the median nerve. It travels deep to the median nerve between the flexor pollicis longus and flexor digitorum profundus (both of which it innervates). The palmar cutaneous branch of the median nerve arises 5 cm proximal to the wrist crease on the radial side of the nerve.[2,3]

Suggested Technique

With ultrasound, the median nerve is usually blocked in the mid-forearm because it is echo-bright without adjacent tendons.[1] This location is also chosen because it is away from the carpal tunnel, proximal to the palmar cutaneous branch takeoff, but distal to the anterior interosseous motor branch takeoff. In the mid-forearm, the median nerve lies within the fascial plane between the flexor digitorum superficialis and profundus, which provides a means for targeting drug injections without nerve contact. The block is performed on the volar side of the forearm with the arm supinated. Both in-plane and out-of-plane approaches can be used for these blocks. Steep in-plane approach to the median nerve from the lateral aspect of the forearm avoids the radial artery and the superficial radial nerve.

The hand should be relaxed so that the median nerve is mobile and not under tension. Wrist hyperextension stretches the median nerve and leads to impairment of nerve function.[4] Therefore, median nerve block should be performed with the wrist in neutral position.

Near the elbow, the median nerve lies medial to the brachial artery. Median nerve block proximal to the elbow is often used in the recovery room following surgery because of the presence of surgical dressings covering the forearm. If this approach is used, care must be taken to avoid puncturing the brachial artery because this can result in median epineurial hematoma.[5,6]

Although the median artery normally evolutes during development, persistent median artery can be detected with high-resolution ultrasound in about 25% of asymptomatic individuals.[7] Persistent median artery is sometimes associated with high division or bifid median nerve, in which cases the artery is often in the middle of the divided nerve. When the persistent median artery is eccentrically located with respect to the nerve, the block should target the nonarterial side of the nerve to avoid intraneural hematoma.

Neurologic Assessment

Sensory block of the median nerve can be tested at the palmar web near the base of the index finger. Motor block of the opponens pollicis can be tested by having the patient touch the base of the small finger with the thumb against resistance. Alternatively, the abductor pollicis brevis can be tested.

References

1. Jamadar DA, Jacobson JA, Hayes CW. Sonographic evaluation of the median nerve at the wrist. *J Ultrasound Med.* 2001;20:1011-1014.
2. Bezerra AJ, Carvalho VC, Nucci A. An anatomical study of the palmar cutaneous branch of the median nerve. *Surg Radiol Anat.* 1986;8:183-188.
3. Tagliafico A, Pugliese F, Bianchi S, et al. High-resolution sonography of the palmar cutaneous branch of the median nerve. *AJR Am J Roentgenol.* 2008;191:107-114.
4. Chowet AL, Lopez JR, Brock-Utne JG, Jaffe RA. Wrist hyperextension leads to median nerve conduction block: implications for intra-arterial catheter placement. *Anesthesiology.* 2004;100:287-291.
5. Macon WL 4th, Futrell JW. Median-nerve neuropathy after percutaneous puncture of the brachial artery in patients receiving anti-coagulants. *N Engl J Med.* 1973;288:1396.
6. Chuang YM, Luo CB, Chou YH, et al. Sonographic diagnosis and treatment of a median nerve epineural hematoma caused by brachial artery catheterization. *J Ultrasound Med.* 2002;21:705-708.
7. Gassner EM, Schocke M, Peer S, et al. Persistent median artery in the carpal tunnel: color Doppler ultrasonographic findings. *J Ultrasound Med.* 2002;21:455-461.

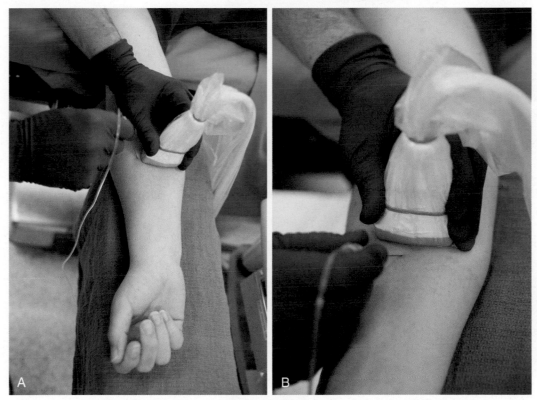

Figure 37-1. External photograph showing the in-plane (**A**) and out-of-plane (**B**) approaches to median nerve block in the forearm. For in-plane technique, the needle approaches from the lateral aspect of the forearm. For out-of-plane technique, the needle approaches from distal to proximal.

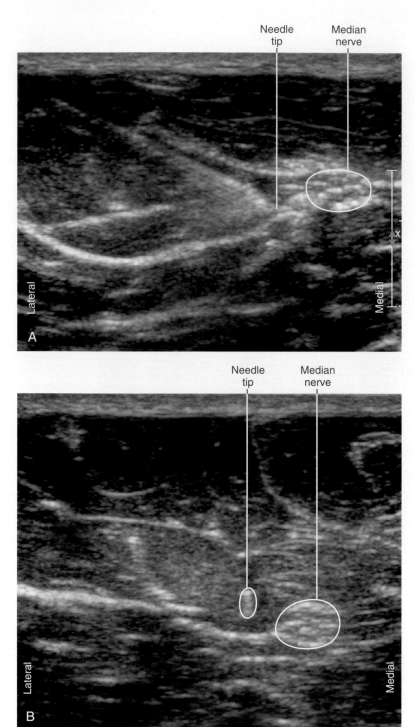

Figure 37-2. Sonograms illustrating the in-plane (**A**) and out-of-plane (**B**) approaches to median nerve block.

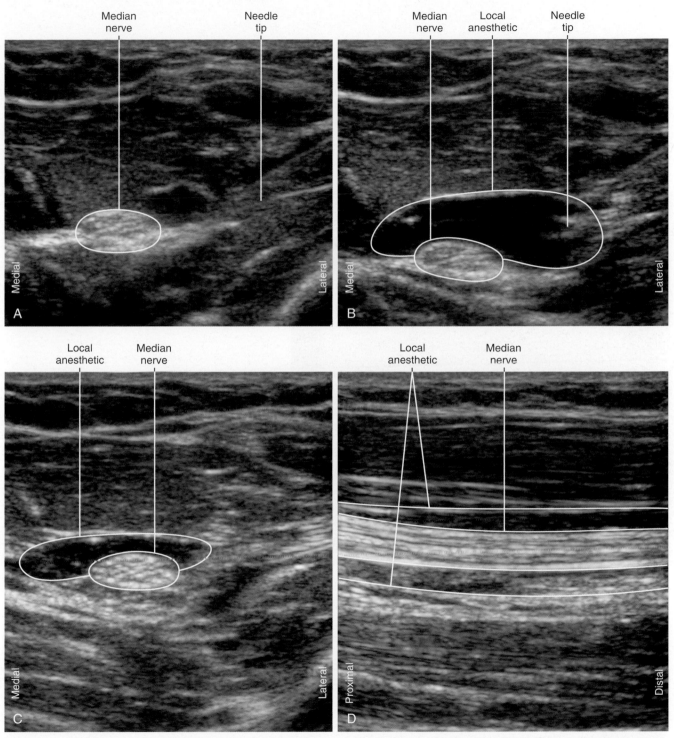

Figure 37-3. Image sequence showing median nerve block in the forearm. An in-plane approach is demonstrated whereby the needle tip is placed between the flexor digitorum superficialis and profundus at the lateral corner of the median nerve (**A** and **B**). Because the local anesthetic is primarily distributed over the surface of the nerve, additional local anesthetic is then deposited underneath the nerve. After completing the injection, local anesthetic is distributed around the median nerve (**C**) and tracks along the nerve (**D**).

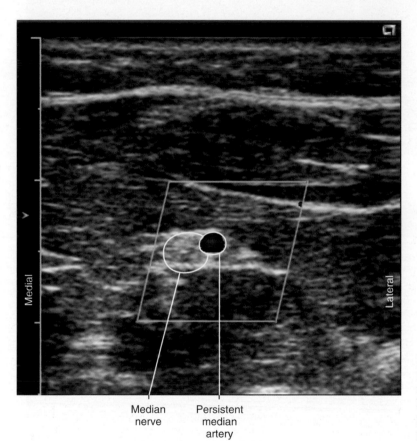

Medial

Lateral

Median   Persistent
nerve   median
              artery

Figure 37-4. A relatively common anatomic variant is persistent median artery. In this variation, the persistent median artery lies within the same connective tissue bundle as the median nerve and can divide it into two parts. When this condition is identified, the needle tip is placed on the side of the nerve away from the artery.

CHAPTER 38

ULNAR NERVE BLOCK

The ulnar nerve is a branch of the medial cord of the brachial plexus. The ulnar nerve provides sensation of the dorsal and palmar sides of the ulnar aspect of the hand. It leaves the neurovascular bundle in the axilla to travel through the cubital tunnel. In the forearm, it joins the ulnar artery on its medial side. The ulnar nerve usually lies between the ulnar artery and the flexor carpi ulnaris (FCU) tendon in the forearm. The dorsal cutaneous branch leaves the ulnar nerve in the forearm proximal to the wrist.[1,2] At the level of the hamate, the ulnar nerve divides into its superficial sensory branch and its deep motor branch.

Suggested Technique

The ulnar nerve is usually blocked just proximal to its juncture with the ulnar artery in the forearm.[3] In this location, the nerve is either oval or triangular. The block is performed with the patient supine and the arm supinated. The needle tip is placed within the fascial plane that connects the ulnar nerve and ulnar artery using an in-plane approach from the lateral side of the forearm. To access this plane with the block needle it is best to puncture the fascia and slowly inject as the needle is pulled back.

A relatively common (3%-10%) anatomic variant is superficial ulnar artery, whereby the ulnar artery lies superficial to the flexor muscles.[4]

Neurologic Assessment

Neurologic assessment of ulnar nerve block includes testing sensation of the ulnar side of the hand. Motor block assessment can be performed by testing the dorsal and palmar interossei functions. These muscles abduct and adduct the fingers, respectively.

References

1. Botte MJ, Cohen MS, Lavernia CJ, et al. The dorsal branch of the ulnar nerve: an anatomic study. *J Hand Surg [Am].* 1990;15:603-607.

2. Grossman JA, Yen L, Rapaport D. The dorsal cutaneous branch of the ulnar nerve: an anatomic clarification with six case reports. *Chir Main.* 1998;17:154-158.
3. Gray AT, Schafhalter-Zoppoth I. Ultrasound guidance for ulnar nerve block in the forearm. *Reg Anesth Pain Med.* 2003; 28:335-339.
4. Schafhalter-Zoppoth I, Gray AT. Ultrasound-guided ulnar nerve block in the presence of a superficial ulnar artery. *Reg Anesth Pain Med.* 2004;29:297-298.

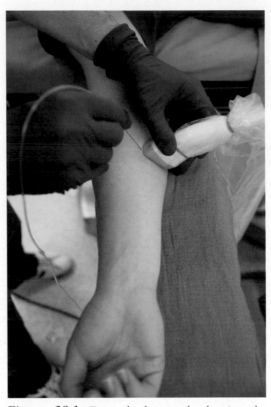

Figure 38-1. External photograph showing the approach to ulnar nerve block in the forearm. An in-plane approach from the lateral aspect of the forearm is shown.

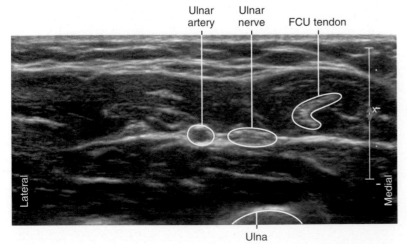

Figure 38-2. Short-axis view of the ulnar nerve in the forearm. The flexor carpi ulnaris (FCU) tendon and ulnar artery are shown. The ulnar nerve normally lies between the FCU tendon and the ulnar artery.

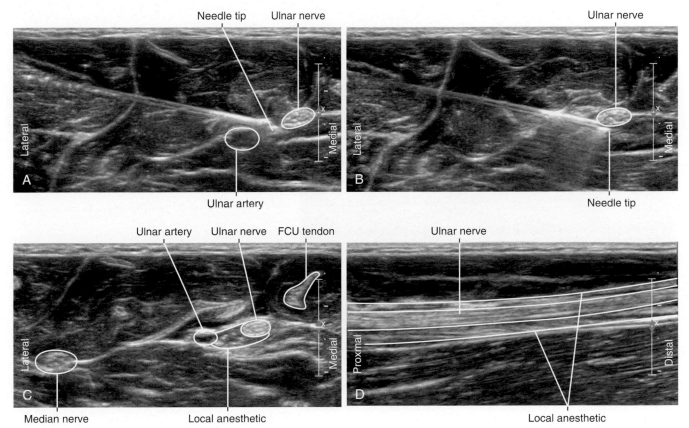

Figure 38-3. Image sequence showing ulnar nerve block in the forearm. An in-plane approach is demonstrated whereby the needle tip is placed between the ulnar artery and ulnar nerve (**A** and **B**). After injection, local anesthetic is distributed around the ulnar nerve (**C**) and tracks along the nerve (**D**).

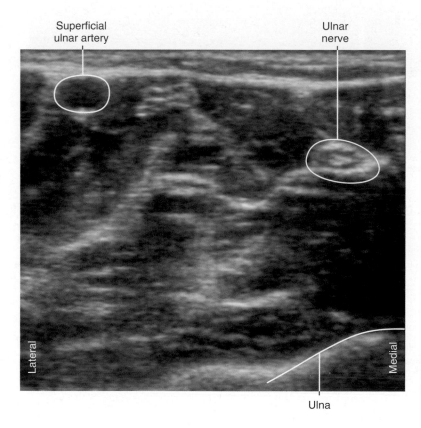

Superficial
ulnar artery

Ulnar
nerve

Lateral

Medial

Ulna

Figure 38-4. A relatively common anatomic variant is superficial ulnar artery. In this variation, the ulnar artery lies superficial to the flexor muscles and is not adjacent to the ulnar nerve.

Lower Extremity Blocks

CHAPTER 39

LATERAL FEMORAL CUTANEOUS NERVE BLOCK

The lateral femoral cutaneous nerve (LFCN) is a sensory nerve derived from the second and third lumbar nerve roots. The nerve is a branch of the lumbar plexus that provides cutaneous sensation from the lateral aspect of the thigh. The nerve emerges from the lumbar plexus to travel across the iliacus muscle and rise up toward the anterior-superior iliac spine (ASIS). The nerve usually enters the anterior thigh medial to the ASIS and then crosses over the sartorius muscle from medial to lateral.

Anatomic variation of the LFCN is common. The nerve may consist of as many as four branches where it exits the pelvis.[1] The nerve passes medial to the ASIS by a variable distance and may cross the pelvic bone to reach the anterior thigh.[2] Rather than passing over the sartorius, in some patients, the LFCN can pass through the sartorius muscle. The estimated incidence of this ranges between 3% and 22%.[3,4] Although the LFCN is referred to as a *discrete nerve*, this designation can indicate a collective set of nerves. Like other cutaneous nerves, the LFCN branches extensively when it enters the subcutaneous tissue. In rare cases (~7%), the LFCN is absent, and its territory is covered by the ilioinguinal and femoral nerves.[3]

High-resolution ultrasound imaging can identify the LFCN superficial to the sartorius muscle in the proximal thigh.[5] The nerve has a characteristic medial to lateral course over this muscle. The nerve and muscle are best visualized just medial and distal to the ASIS. As with other small nerves, it is necessary to scan along the length of the nerve to confirm nerve identity. The best imaging technique is to slide the transducer along the known course of the nerve with the nerve viewed in short axis. LFCNs that pass through the sartorius are easier to image because the nerve is surrounded by hypoechoic muscle that provides better acoustic contrast than echobright subcutaneous tissue. Although ultrasound imaging of the LFCN has been reported,[6] the nerve is normally small (1-3 mm in diameter), and sonographic visualization can be difficult within the echobright subcutaneous tissue of the anterior thigh.

LFCN block can be used alone or in conjunction with other lower extremity blocks. It is useful for skin graft harvests and surgical procedures with lateral incisions of the thigh. It is one of the few lower extremity blocks for weight-bearing patients (this group also includes ankle block and saphenous block). LFCN block can improve thigh tourniquet tolerance when combined with other lower extremity blocks.[7]

If adequate volume is administered, separate LFCN block is not normally necessary after ultrasound-guided femoral block. However, as volume reduction for femoral blocks becomes more feasible because of more targeted injections, sparing of the other nerves such as the LFCN will occur.

Ultrasound imaging may be useful for the diagnosis and treatment of meralgia paresthetica (from Greek *meros* for "thigh," and *algos* for "pain"). Meralgia can result from mechanical stretch or compression injury of the LFCN. Abnormal nerve morphology has been described in patients with meralgia paresthetica. Fusiform enlargement of the LFCN, loss of fascicular discrimination, and hyperemia can all occur in this condition.[8,9]

Suggested Technique

LFCN blocks are performed in the supine position. The sartorius muscle is imaged in short-axis view near its insertion on the ASIS. By sliding the ultrasound transducer back and forth between proximal and distal locations, the LFCN is identified by its characteristic lateral course over the sartorius muscle. The in-plane approach can be used from the lateral aspect of the thigh. Acoustic standoff may be advantageous in thin patients to image the LFCN close to the ASIS, so that the conforming gel pad forms around the bone.

It may not be critical to directly visualize the LFCN for block success. When the nerve is not sonographically visible, our recommendation for performing LFCN block is to image the sartorius muscle in short-axis view near the ASIS. The sartorius muscle has a triangular or circular shape near its origin on the ASIS. The fascial planes that lie over the anterior border of the sartorius muscle (in particular, the fascia lata) can be separated by infiltrating local anesthetic between layers.

Clinical Pearls

- The LFCN can be imaged between the fascia iliaca and the fascia lata. If light probe pressure is applied, the nerve can be seen within the tissue between these two fascial layers for needle tip placement.[10]
- LFCN block is assessed by cutaneous anesthesia midway between the ASIS and the lateral knee joint line.[11]
- In some patients, the crossing of the LFCN with the deep circumflex iliac artery can be identified on sagittal oblique sonograms.[12] This view is parallel to the course of the nerve and perpendicular to the course of the artery.

References

1. Surucu HS, Tanyeli E, Sargon MF, Karahan ST. An anatomic study of the lateral femoral cutaneous nerve. *Surg Radiol Anat.* 1997;19:307-310.
2. Hospodar PP, Ashman ES, Traub JA. Anatomic study of the lateral femoral cutaneous nerve with respect to the ilioinguinal surgical dissection. *J Orthop Trauma.* 1999;13:17-19.
3. de Ridder VA, de Lange S, Popta JV. Anatomical variations of the lateral femoral cutaneous nerve and the consequences for surgery. *J Orthop Trauma.* 1999;13:207-211.
4. Dias Filho LC, Valenca MM, Guimaraes Filho FA, et al. Lateral femoral cutaneous neuralgia: an anatomical insight. *Clin Anat.* 2003;16:309-316.
5. Thain LM, Downey DB. Sonography of peripheral nerves: technique, anatomy, and pathology. *Ultrasound Q.* 2002;18:225-245.
6. Van Holsbeeck M, Introcaso JH, eds. *Musculoskeletal Ultrasound*, 2nd ed. St. Louis: Mosby; 2001.
7. Morin AM, Pandurovic M, Eberhart LH, et al. Is a blockade of the lateral cutaneous nerve of the thigh an alternative to the classical femoral nerve blockade for knee joint arthroscopy? A randomised controlled study. *Anaesthesist* 2005;54:991-999.

8. Hurdle MF, Weingarten TN, Crisostomo RA, et al. Ultrasound-guided blockade of the lateral femoral cutaneous nerve: technical description and review of 10 cases. *Arch Phys Med Rehabil*. 2007;88:1362-1364.

9. Tumber PS, Bhatia A, Chan VW. Ultrasound-guided lateral femoral cutaneous nerve block for meralgia paresthetica. *Anesth Analg*. 2008;106:1021-1022.

10. Ng I, Vaghadia H, Choi PT, Helmy N. Ultrasound imaging accurately identifies the lateral femoral cutaneous nerve. *Anesth Analg*. 2008;107:1070-1074.

11. Shannon J, Lang SA, Yip RW, Gerard M. Lateral femoral cutaneous nerve block revisited. A nerve stimulator technique. *Reg Anesth*. 1995;20:100-104.

12. Damarey B, Demondion X, Boutry N, et al. Sonographic assessment of the lateral femoral cutaneous nerve. *J Clin Ultrasound*. 2009;37:89-95.

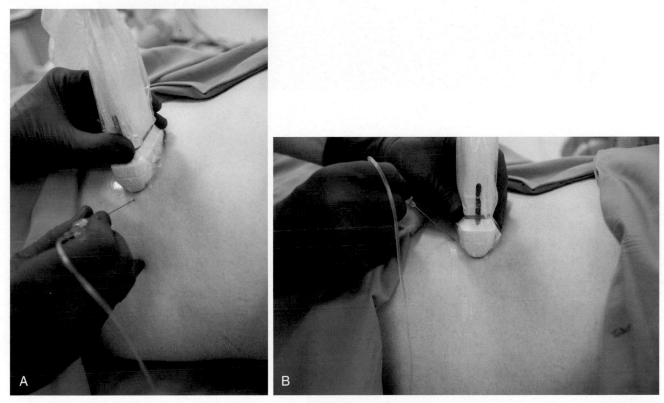

Figure 39-1. External photograph showing the approaches to lateral femoral cutaneous nerve block. An in-plane approach from the lateral aspect of the thigh is shown (**A**). An out-of-plane approach from distal to proximal is shown (**B**).

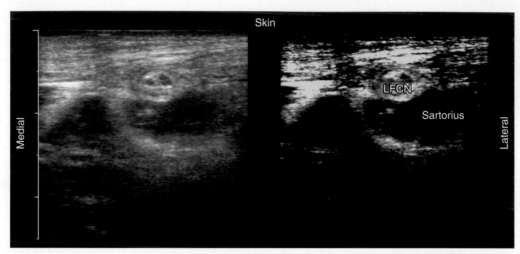

Figure 39-2. Short-axis view of the LFCN over the sartorius muscle near its proximal insertion on the ASIS. This large bifascicular nerve will divide more distally in the thigh.

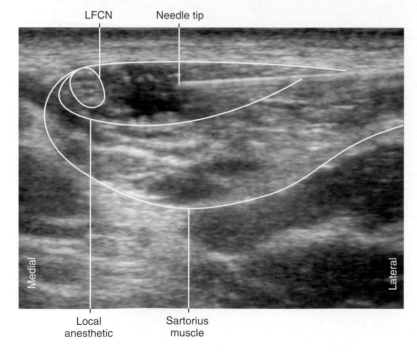

Figure 39-3. Needle tip in place for injection of local anesthetic for in-plane LFCN block. In this example, the nerve is pushed against the sartorius muscle.

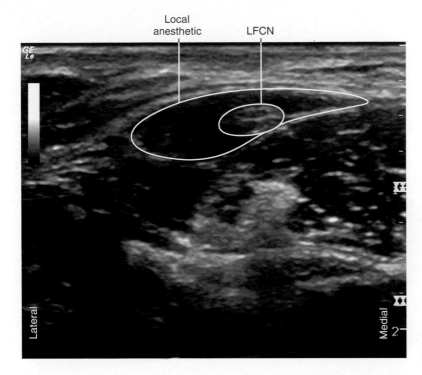

Figure 39-4. An in-plane approach demonstrates local anesthetic distributed around a fascicular LFCN nerve.

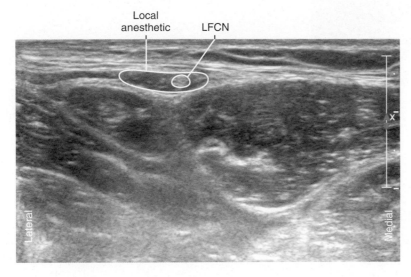

Figure 39-5. After injection, local anesthetic is seen to surround the LFCN.

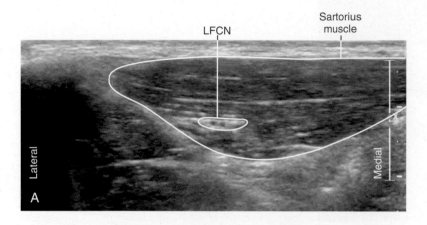

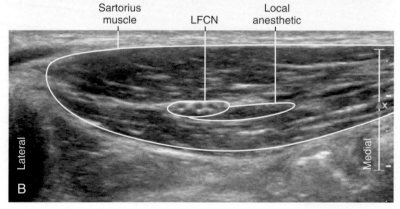

Figure 39-6. Pass-through LFCN. In this anatomic variation, the LFCN passes through the sartorius muscle rather than over it. Although relatively uncommon, this variant is easily recognized. The nerve is shown before (**A**) and after (**B**) injection of local anesthetic.

CHAPTER 40

FEMORAL NERVE BLOCK

The femoral nerve is the largest branch of the lumbar plexus. It provides motor innervation to the quadriceps, sartorius, and pectineus muscles. The sensory branches include the anterior cutaneous nerve of the thigh, the infrapatellar nerve, and the saphenous nerve. These nerves innervate the anterior thigh, the patella, and the medial leg and foot, respectively.

The normal femoral nerve is oval or triangular in cross section, with dimensions of about 3 mm in anteroposterior diameter and 10 mm in mediolateral diameter in the inguinal region.[1] The femoral nerve usually lies lateral to the femoral artery but can contact or lie underneath the femoral artery in 15% of cases. In about one third of individuals, the femoral nerve is triangular in the suprainguinal region on short-axis scans.

The femoral nerve is covered by echogenic subcutaneous tissue and fascia. The nerve lies on the hypoechoic iliopsoas muscle, which has a characteristic medial-lateral inclination. This incline positions the lateral side of the nerve slightly closer to the skin surface. At this interface of bright fascia and dark muscle, the nerve can be difficult to visualize. The best nerve visibility is proximal to the inguinal crease before the femoral nerve and femoral artery divide into smaller branches distally. In this proximal location, the femoral nerve puts a small dent in the shape of the iliopsoas muscle. This occurs because the femoral nerve lies in the groove between the iliacus and psoas components of the muscle. The tilt of the transducer strongly influences femoral nerve visibility owing to anisotropic effects.[2] With ultrasound guidance, it may be possible to perform more proximal drug injections and therefore more complete resultant femoral nerve blocks.

Suggested Technique

Femoral nerve block is performed in the supine position with the nerve viewed in short axis. The lateral corner of the nerve is targeted to avoid the femoral vessels and to make the injection closest to the skin surface. Both out-of-plane (from distal to proximal) and in-plane (from lateral to medial) approaches can be used. It is critical that the needle tip be positioned between the fascia iliaca and iliopsoas muscle.[3] It is not important to position the needle tip immediately adjacent to the nerve.

The needle tip should be placed in the layer under the femoral nerve so that the injection lifts the nerve toward the surface. This is especially important when catheters are placed. Successful injections not only surround the femoral nerve but also track along its small distal branches. If there is any concern that the injection has not surrounded the femoral nerve, the distal tracking of local anesthetic can be verified by sliding the transducer along the nerve path. If local anesthetic appears to layer only over the femoral nerve, be concerned the fascia iliaca is still intact.

Dull block needles can be used to detect tissue layers, both by visual inspection of the tent and recoil with needle advancement and by tactile sense. If sharp needles are used, the operator's hand motion and needle tip position will be more closely correlated. It may be necessary to combine ultrasound and nerve stimulation for femoral nerve blocks in morbidly obese patients. In these patients, the femoral artery can be imaged to give an approximate location for nerve stimulation.

Posterior acoustic enhancement occurs deep to the femoral artery.[4] This artifact should not be confused with the femoral nerve. The femoral nerve and iliopsoas tendon can be distinguished because the iliopsoas tendon normally lies deep within the iliopsoas muscle.

The lateral to medial in-plane approach to femoral block has potential disadvantages because of the longer needle path, which can be near the lateral femoral cutaneous nerve. In addition, the needle has a tendency to skim along the fascia iliaca, deforming it rather than puncturing it. This can be particularly frustrating as the needle tip approaches the femoral artery.

Many institutions have found the out-of-plane approach to be very safe and effective.[5] However, the operator must be cognizant of the unimaged needle path. Branches of the femoral artery may potentially lie within the unimaged needle path short of the scan plane.[6] Scanning before needle placement can be advantageous.

The incidence of vascular puncture rates with nerve stimulation–guided femoral nerve catheters is about 6%.[7] Ultrasound guidance likely reduces that incidence. Puncture of the inguinal vessels can result in blood tracking into the retroperitoneum, even if the puncture occurs distal to the inguinal ligament.[8]

Clinical Pearls

- Some clinicians advocate an oblique out-of-plane approach to femoral nerve block.[9] This approach from the lateral aspect of the thigh allows needle tip placement under the posterior aspect of the nerve. The needle tip punctures the fascia iliaca at the lateral corner of the femoral nerve.
- The iliopsoas tendon lies under the femoral artery and should not be mistaken for the femoral nerve.[10]
- Transducer location is of paramount importance to femoral nerve visibility. If the transducer is too distal, the nerve and artery will divide. This will compromise nerve visibility because it is difficult to image small femoral nerve branches, particularly those that branch to the surface, within the echobright subcutaneous tissue (only after injection of anechoic fluid can these branches be seen). If the transducer is too proximal, the nerve and artery will dive away from the transducer on the surface on the iliacus muscle.

References

1. Gruber H, Peer S, Kovacs P, et al. The ultrasonographic appearance of the femoral nerve and cases of iatrogenic impairment. *J Ultrasound Med.* 2003;22:163-172.
2. Soong J, Schafhalter-Zoppoth I, Gray AT. The importance of transducer angle to ultrasound visibility of the femoral nerve. *Reg Anesth Pain Med.* 2005;30:505.
3. Dalens B, Vanneuville G, Tanguy A. Comparison of the fascia iliaca compartment block with the 3-in-1 block in children. *Anesth Analg.* 1989;69:705-713.
4. Filly RA, Sommer FG, Minton MJ. Characterization of biological fluids by ultrasound and computed tomography. *Radiology.* 1980;134:167-171.

5. Sites BD, Spence BC, Gallagher JD, et al. Characterizing novice behavior associated with learning ultrasound-guided peripheral regional anesthesia. *Reg Anesth Pain Med.* 2007;32:107-115.
6. Orebaugh SL. The femoral nerve and its relationship to the lateral circumflex femoral artery. *Anesth Analg.* 2006;102:1859-1862.
7. Wiegel M, Gottschaldt U, Hennebach R, et al. Complications and adverse effects associated with continuous peripheral nerve blocks in orthopedic patients. *Anesth Analg.* 2007;104:1578-1582.
8. Spies JB, Berlin L. Complications of femoral artery puncture. *AJR Am J Roentgenol.* 1998;170:9-11.
9. Fredrickson M. "Oblique" needle-probe alignment to facilitate ultrasound-guided femoral catheter placement. *Reg Anesth Pain Med.* 2008;33:383-384.
10. Mulroy RD. The iliopsoas muscle complex: iliacus muscle, psoas tendon release. *Clin Orthop.* 1965;38:81-85.

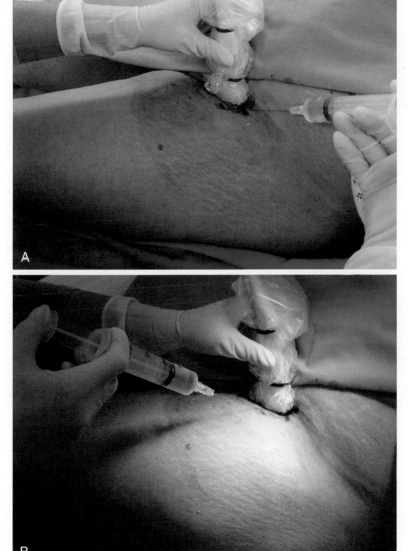

Figure 40-1. External photograph showing approaches to femoral nerve block in the inguinal region. An in-plane approach from the lateral aspect of the thigh is shown (**A**). An out-of-plane approach is also shown (**B**).

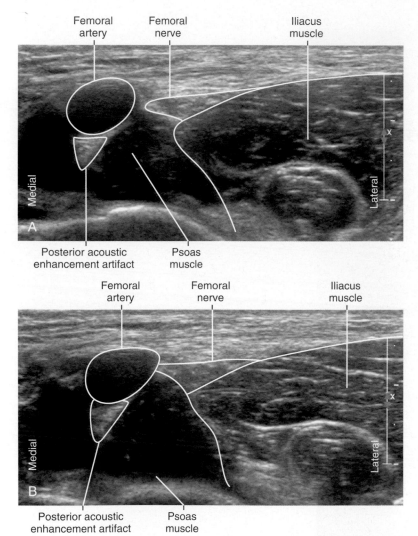

Figure 40-2. Short-axis views of the femoral nerve in the inguinal region. The inclination of the transducer is critical to visibility of the femoral nerve (**A** and **B**). In this example, the echoes from a triangular femoral nerve disappear when the transducer is tilted (the property of *anisotropy*).

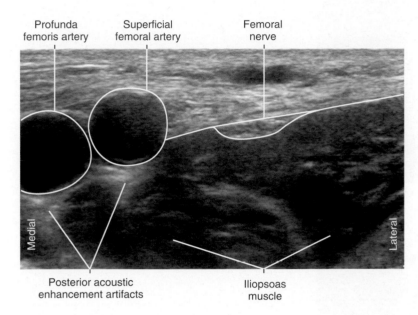

Profunda femoris artery

Superficial femoral artery

Femoral nerve

Medial

Lateral

Posterior acoustic enhancement artifacts

Iliopsoas muscle

Figure 40-3. Short-axis view of the femoral nerve in the inguinal region. In this example, the femoral nerve appears to indent the iliopsoas muscle. Ultrasound visibility of the femoral nerve is complicated by the fact that the nerve lies at the interface of hyperechoic subcutaneous tissue and hypoechoic muscle. In this sonogram, the femoral artery has divided into its superficial and profunda branches.

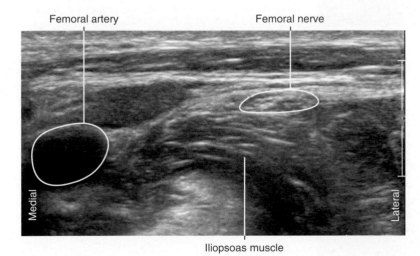

Femoral artery

Femoral nerve

Medial

Lateral

Iliopsoas muscle

Figure 40-4. Short-axis view of the femoral nerve in the proximal inguinal region. In this example, the femoral nerve appears far lateral from the femoral artery.

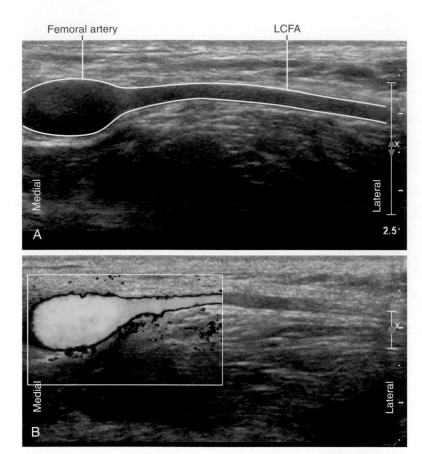

Figure 40-5. The femoral artery is seen in short-axis view with the lateral circumflex femoral artery in long-axis view (**A**). A duplex image is shown with power Doppler verifying color encoding of the vessels (**B**).

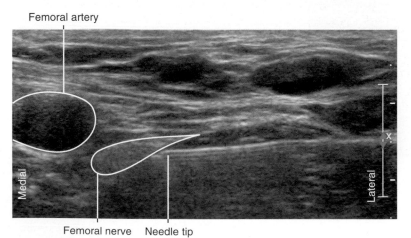

Figure 40-6. Short-axis in-plane approach to femoral nerve block. The needle tip approaches the femoral nerve from the lateral side.

Femoral artery   Femoral nerve

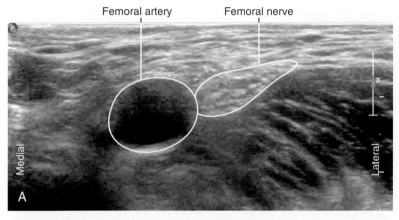

Femoral artery   Local anesthetic

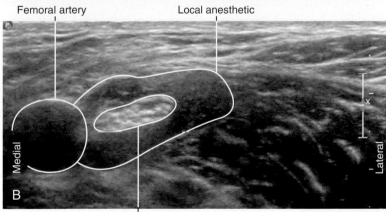

Femoral nerve

Figure 40-7. Femoral nerve visibility before (**A**) and after (**B**) injection of local anesthetic. The nerve visibility is improved by posterior acoustic enhancement. This femoral nerve is oval.

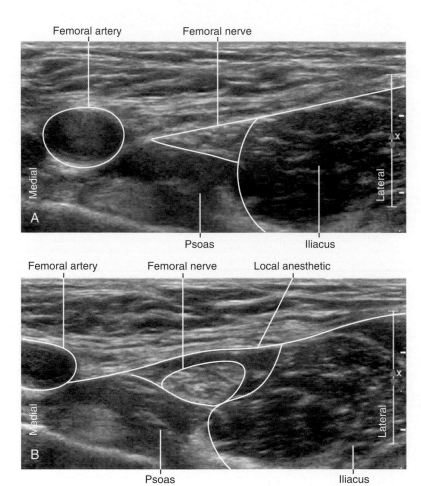

Figure 40-8. Femoral nerve in short-axis view before (**A**) and after (**B**) injection of local anesthetic. In this example, a triangular femoral nerve is observed to lie in the groove between the iliacus and psoas muscles. After injection, branching of the nerve is observed in a slightly more distal location.

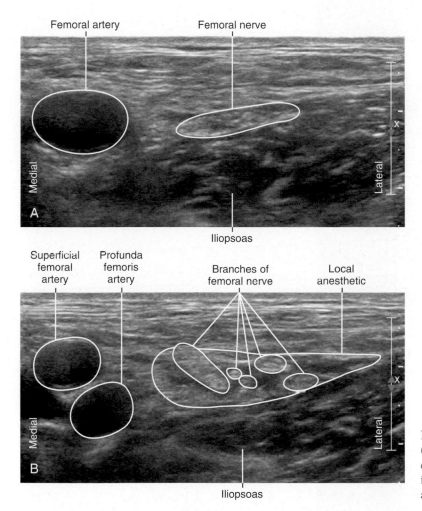

Femoral artery   Femoral nerve

Medial

Lateral

A

Iliopsoas

Superficial   Profunda
femoral   femoris
artery   artery   Branches of   Local
                                     femoral nerve   anesthetic

Medial

Lateral

B

Iliopsoas

Figure 40-9. Femoral nerve in short-axis view before (**A**) and after (**B**) injection of local anesthetic. In this example, small branches of the femoral nerve are seen after injection of local anesthetic. This tracking pattern of local anesthetic verifies successful block.

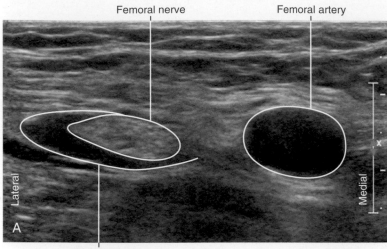

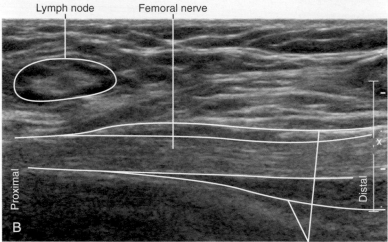

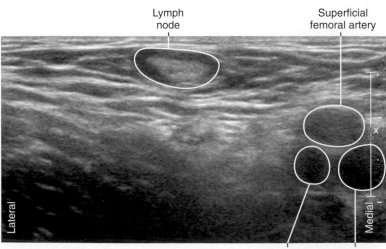

Figure 40-10. Femoral nerve in short-axis (**A**) and long-axis (**B**) views after injection of local anesthetic. Local anesthetic is distributed around the femoral nerve (**A**) and tracks along the nerve (**B**).

Figure 40-11. An inguinal lymph node observed during femoral nerve block.

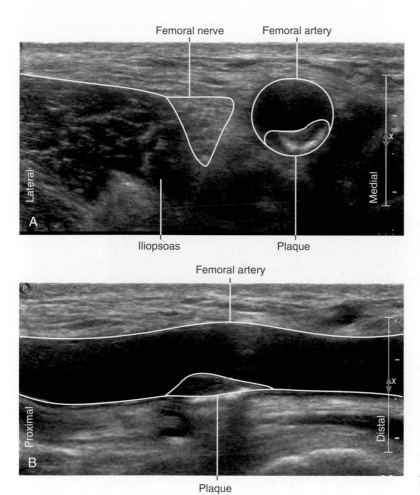

Femoral nerve   Femoral artery

Lateral

Medial

A

Iliopsoas   Plaque

Femoral artery

Proximal

Distal

B

Plaque

Figure 40-12. Femoral artery plaque observed in short-axis (**A**) and long-axis (**B**) views during femoral nerve block.

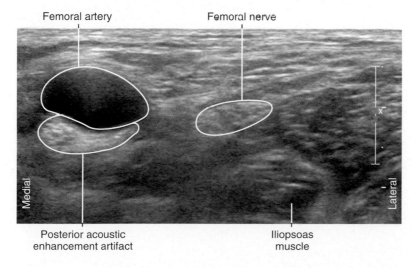

Femoral artery   Femoral nerve

Medial

Lateral

Posterior acoustic
enhancement artifact

Iliopsoas
muscle

Figure 40-13. Posterior acoustic enhancement of echoes deep to the femoral artery. In this example, the artifact has similar echotexture to a peripheral nerve.

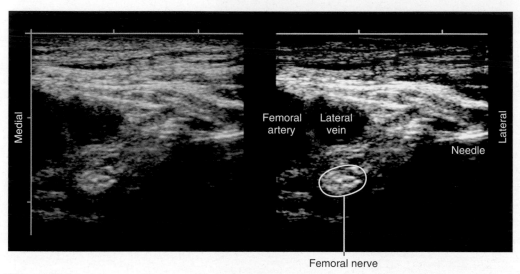

Figure 40-14. Anatomic variation in the inguinal region. In this example, the femoral nerve is observed deep to an accessory lateral femoral vein.

CHAPTER 41

SAPHENOUS NERVE BLOCK

The saphenous nerve is a sensory branch of the femoral nerve that travels with the femoral artery in the thigh along with the infrapatellar nerve and a nerve to the vastus medialis.[1] Under the sartorius muscle, this complex forms the subsartorial plexus, which also can include contributions from the posterior division of the obturator nerve.[2] The femoral artery and these nerves separate at the entrance to the adductor canal.[3,4]

The saphenous nerve emerges into the subcutaneous tissue between the sartorius and gracilis tendons within the pes anserinus to join the undersurface of the saphenous vein near the knee crease. The saphenous nerve and vein travel together in the leg to lie anterior to the medial malleolus. Saphenous nerve block is important for surgical anesthesia of the foot and ankle because it innervates the medial leg, malleolus, and foot. There are many approaches to saphenous nerve block along the course of the nerve.[5]

Suggested Technique

Subsartorial Plexus Block (Mid-Thigh)

Saphenous nerve block can be performed in the mid-thigh with the patient in the supine position. An in-plane approach from the anterior thigh can be used to direct the needle tip through the sartorius muscle. The nerves of the subsartorial plexus can be imaged as a "bright triangle" anterior to the femoral artery. The needle tip crosses the fascial plane on the anterior side of the nerves to avoid the neurovascular bundle. This subsartorial saphenous block is the deepest saphenous nerve block and therefore requires a steep angle of approach. However, the subsartorial plexus can often be directly imaged with ultrasound. The best access to the fascial layer of the nerves of the subsartorial plexus is usually attained by passing the block needle through the sartorius muscle rather than the vastus medialis. This trans-sartorial approach is similar to previous descriptions of saphenous nerve block that involved nerve stimulation.[6]

Vastoadductor Membrane Block (Distal Thigh)

Saphenous nerve block also can be performed in the distal thigh with the patient in the supine position.[7] An in-plane approach can be used to direct the needle tip through the vastus medialis just adjacent to the sartorius muscle. The muscles are viewed in short axis by placing the transducer on the distal aspect of the medial thigh with the needle introduced anteriorly. The local anesthetic injection should track within the fascial plane deep to the sartorius. Direct imaging of the saphenous nerve and the accompanying branch of the femoral artery is sometimes possible within this fascial plane.

Subcutaneous Infiltration Block (Proximal Leg)

Saphenous nerve block can also be performed in the leg at the level of the tibial tuberosity.[8] For this procedure, local anesthetic is infiltrated within the subcutaneous tissue near the saphenous vein using either an in-plane or out-of-plane approach. At this level, the saphenous nerve and saphenous vein both lie superficial to the fascia lata. If the saphenous vein is difficult to visualize, a proximal tourniquet can be applied.

Clinical Pearls

- The saphenous nerve is a branch of the posterior division of the femoral nerve.
- The relation of the saphenous nerve to the femoral artery changes from lateral (near the inguinal region) to anterior (in the adductor canal).
- For the mid-thigh approach to saphenous nerve block, the sartorius muscle should be placed on the edge of the screen in short-axis view so that the block needle will traverse this muscle for injection underneath it.
- This approach is similar to the subsartorial approach to saphenous nerve block.[6]
- Rotate the leg to improve the sartorial coverage of the saphenous nerve complex. This will place the needle path through this muscle rather than the vastus medialis. Needle placement through the vastus medialis is more uncomfortable for the patient and more difficult for access to the fascial layers containing the nerves.
- After the injection under the sartorius muscle, slide the transducer over the known course of the saphenous nerve to verify the local anesthetic tracks along the branches of the subsartorial plexus.
- More distal block of the saphenous nerve is potentially more selective and carries less risk for vascular puncture. However, direct nerve imaging can be difficult with these distal approaches.

References

1. Thiranagama R. Nerve supply of the human vastus medialis muscle. *J Anat*. 1990;170:193-198.
2. Bouaziz H, Vial F, Jochum D, et al. An evaluation of the cutaneous distribution after obturator nerve block. *Anesth Analg*. 2002;94:445-449.
3. Scholten FG, Mali WP, Hillen B, van Leeuwen MS. US location of the adductor canal hiatus: morphologic study. *Radiology*. 1989;172:75-78.
4. Tubbs RS, Loukas M, Shoja MM, et al. Anatomy and potential clinical significance of the vastoadductor membrane. *Surg Radiol Anat*. 2007;29:569-573.

5. Benzon HT, Sharma S, Calimaran A. Comparison of the different approaches to saphenous nerve block. *Anesthesiology.* 2005;102:633-638.
6. Mansour NY. Sub-sartorial saphenous nerve block with the aid of nerve stimulator. *Reg Anesth.* 1993;18:266-268.
7. Krombach J, Gray AT. Sonography for saphenous nerve block near the adductor canal. *Reg Anesth Pain Med.* 2007;32:369-370.
8. Gray AT, Collins AB. Ultrasound-guided saphenous nerve block. *Reg Anesth Pain Med.* 2003;28:148.

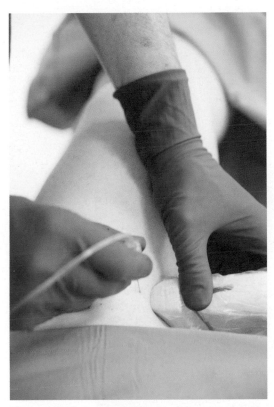

Figure 41-1. External photograph showing the sub-sartorial approach to saphenous nerve block in the mid-thigh. An in-plane approach from the anterior aspect of the thigh is shown.

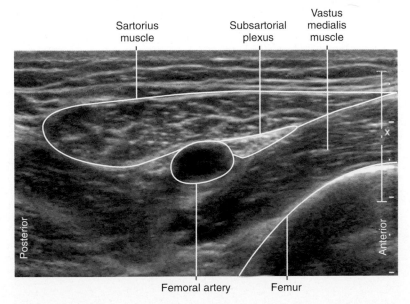

Figure 41-2. Short-axis view of the sartorius muscle, femoral artery, and subsartorial plexus in the mid-thigh. The femoral vein has been compressed by the ultrasound transducer.

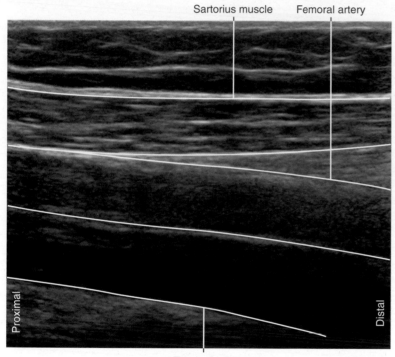

Sartorius muscle   Femoral artery

Proximal

Distal

Femoral vein

Figure 41-3. Long-axis view of the femoral artery and vein underneath the sartorius muscle in the mid-thigh. The subsartorial block of the saphenous nerve is usually performed where the femoral artery is in contact with the sartorius muscle before it leaves into the adductor canal.

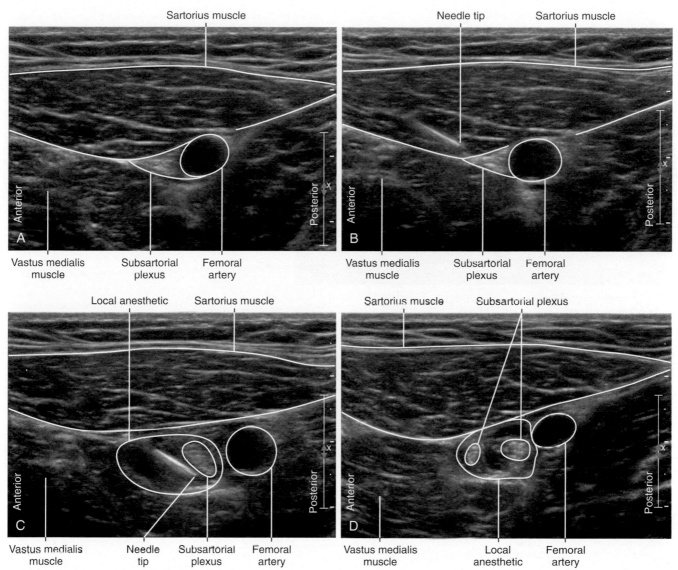

Sartorius muscle

Needle tip   Sartorius muscle

Anterior

Posterior

A

Anterior

Posterior

B

Vastus medialis
muscle

Subsartorial
plexus

Femoral
artery

Vastus medialis
muscle

Subsartorial
plexus

Femoral
artery

Local anesthetic   Sartorius muscle

Sartorius muscle   Subsartorial plexus

Anterior

Posterior

C

Anterior

Posterior

D

Vastus medialis
muscle

Needle
tip

Subsartorial
plexus

Femoral
artery

Vastus medialis
muscle

Local
anesthetic

Femoral
artery

Figure 41-4. Image sequence showing subsartorial block of the saphenous nerve in the mid-thigh. The sartorius muscle and subsartorial plexus are imaged in short-axis view (**A**). An in-plane approach is demonstrated whereby the needle tip is placed through the sartorius muscle, targeting the fascial plane on the anterior side of the femoral artery (**B** and **C**). After injection, local anesthetic is distributed around two nerves under the sartorius muscle (**D**).

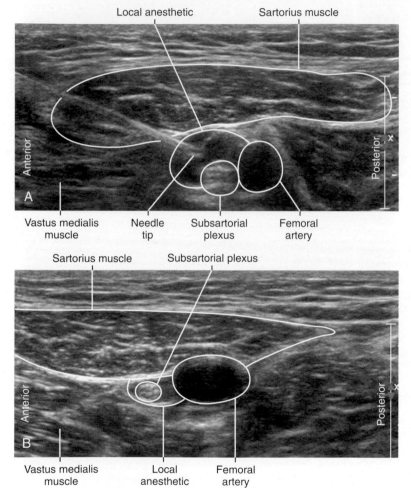

A

Local anesthetic

Sartorius muscle

Anterior

Posterior

Vastus medialis muscle

Needle tip

Subsartorial plexus

Femoral artery

B

Sartorius muscle

Subsartorial plexus

Anterior

Posterior

Vastus medialis muscle

Local anesthetic

Femoral artery

Figure 41-5. Image sequence showing subsartorial block of the saphenous nerve in the mid-thigh with the sartorius muscle and subsartorial plexus imaged in short-axis view. An in-plane approach is demonstrated whereby the needle tip is placed through the sartorius muscle, targeting the fascial plane on the anterior side of the femoral artery (**A**). In this example, after injection, the local anesthetic is distributed around a single nerve complex underneath the sartorius muscle (**B**).

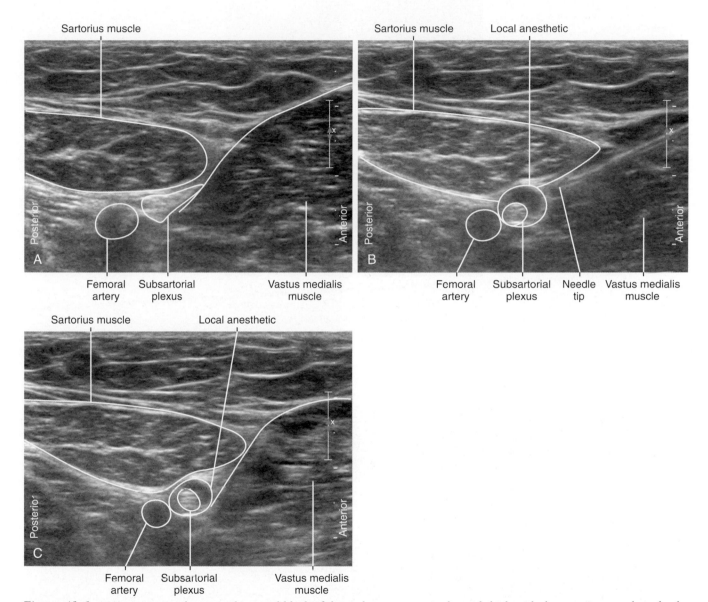

Figure 41-6. Image sequence showing subsartorial block of the saphenous nerve in the mid-thigh with the sartorius muscle and subsartorial plexus imaged in short-axis view (**A**). An in-plane approach is demonstrated whereby the needle tip is placed through the vastus medialis muscle, targeting the nerves on the anterior side of the femoral artery (**B**). In this example, after injection, the local anesthetic is distributed around a single nerve complex underneath the sartorius muscle (**C**).

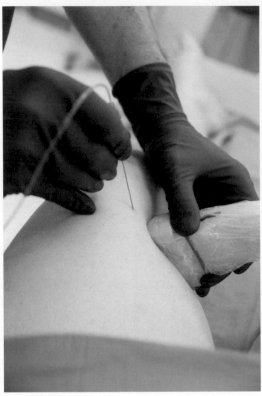

Figure 41-7. External photograph showing the approach to saphenous nerve block in the distal thigh. An in-plane approach from the anterior aspect of the thigh is shown.

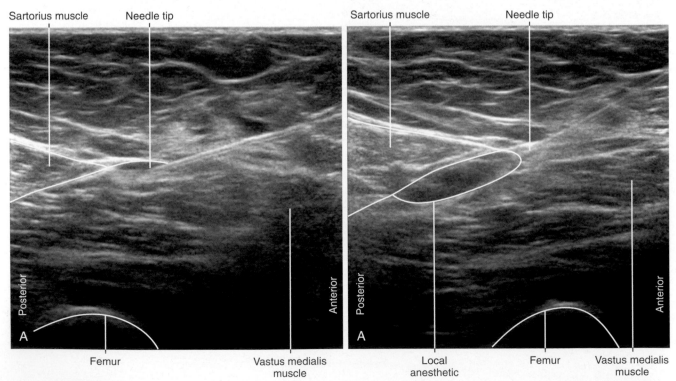

Figure 41-8. Image sequence showing block of the saphenous nerve in the distal thigh. Before injection, the plane between the vastus medialis and sartorius is imaged (**A**). After injection, the local anesthetic divides this fascial plane that contains the saphenous nerve (**B**).

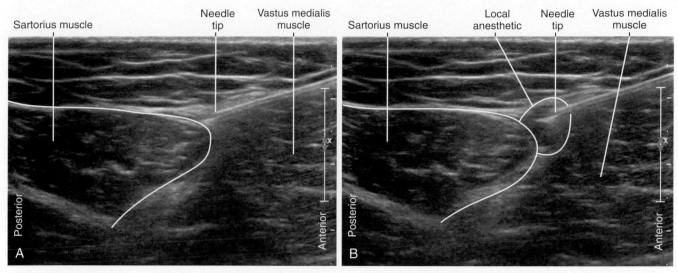

Figure 41-9. Image sequence showing block of the saphenous nerve in the distal thigh. In this example, the superficial aspect of the fascial plane between the vastus medialis and the sartorius muscle is targeted (**A** and **B**).

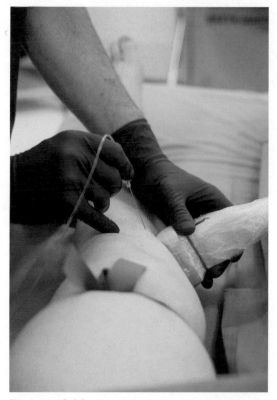

Figure 41-10. External photograph showing the approach to saphenous nerve block in the proximal leg. An in-plane approach from the anterior aspect of the leg is shown. A thigh tourniquet has been applied to distend the saphenous vein to improve its visibility. The saphenous vein is joined by the saphenous nerve in this location.

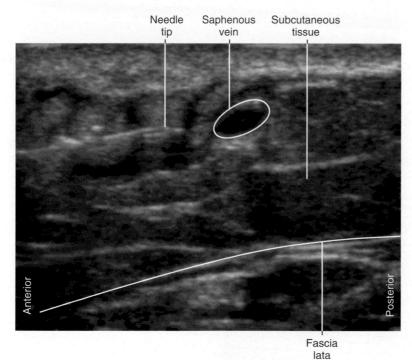

Figure 41-11. Sonogram illustrating infiltration of local anesthetic around the saphenous vein within the subcutaneous tissue of the proximal leg. An in-plane approach from the anterior aspect of the leg is shown.

CHAPTER 42

OBTURATOR NERVE BLOCK

The obturator nerve arises from the lumbar plexus and innervates most of the adductors of the medial compartment of the thigh. The other adductors are the pectineus (innervated by the femoral nerve) and the adductor magnus (partially innervated by the sciatic nerve). The abundance of motor fibers makes the obturator nerve a frequent choice for electromyographic (EMG) recording of compound motor action potentials (CMAPs).[1]

The cutaneous innervation by the obturator nerve is variable.[2] However, there are morphine-sparing effects of obturator nerve block after major surgical procedures. In blocks in which multiple nerves of the lower extremity are targeted (e.g., the posterior lumbar plexus block or the anterior 3-in-1 block), the obturator nerve has a relatively low block success rate. Therefore, obturator nerve block is an important adjunct for lower extremity analgesia. Other indications for obturator nerve block include relief of hip pain, treatment of adductor spasticity, and prevention of obturator stimulation during transurethral resection of lateral bladder wall tumors. Change in adductor strength is the best method for assessing obturator nerve block. However, even with complete obturator nerve block, there is some residual adductor strength because of the pectineus (femoral nerve innervation) and part of the adductor magnus (sciatic nerve innervation) muscles.

Suggested Technique

The anterior and posterior divisions of the obturator nerve converge proximally along the lateral border of the adductor brevis muscle. The obturator nerve divisions are thin and flat as the fascicles disperse to the muscle groups. The obturator nerve divisions have the "white bands" appearance on sonography.[3] It is important that the flat surfaces of the obturator nerve divisions are perpendicular to the sound beam to enhance their echo brightness. Note that although the anterior and posterior divisions converge along the lateral border of the adductor brevis, they do not actually meet there in most (75%-80%) subjects because the divisions remain separated by the obturator externus muscle.[4] Therefore, the obturator nerve block is performed as a multiple-injection technique targeting each of the two divisions separately.

The block is performed in supine position with the leg slightly abducted. The obturator divisions and adductor brevis are visualized in short-axis view in the medial thigh. This is best accomplished by sliding the transducer between proximal and distal locations to observe the convergence of the divisions along the lateral border of the adductor brevis. An out-of-plane approach is often used because of the proximity of the femoral vessels to the unimaged needle path for an in-plane approach. The block is usually performed where the anterior and posterior divisions are just separated by the adductor brevis, with the deeper posterior division targeted first. The local anesthetic distribution should be within the fascia that invests the adductor brevis and the obturator divisions. If the obturator nerve divisions cannot be visualized, a trans–adductor brevis injection can be performed. Care is taken to avoid puncture of the adjacent obturator arteries because puncture of these vessels can cause hemorrhage.[5]

Clinical Pearls

- An accessory obturator nerve is present in about 8.7% of subjects.[6] When present, this nerve partially contributes to motor innervation of the pectineus.
- In some patients, branches entering the adductor brevis can be visualized, giving the appearance of three divisions to the obturator nerve. Position of the obturator arteries with respect to the obturator divisions is variable.

References

1. Atanassoff PG, Weiss BM, Brull SJ, et al. Compound motor action potential recording distinguishes differential onset of motor block of the obturator nerve in response to etidocaine or bupivacaine. *Anesth Analg.* 1996;82:317-320.
2. Bouaziz H, Vial F, Jochum D, et al. An evaluation of the cutaneous distribution after obturator nerve block. *Anesth Analg.* 2002;94:445-449.
3. Soong J, Schafhalter-Zoppoth I, Gray AT. Sonographic imaging of the obturator nerve for regional block. *Reg Anesth Pain Med.* 2007;32:146-151.
4. Choquet O, Capdevila X, Bennourine K, et al. A new inguinal approach for the obturator nerve block: anatomical and randomized clinical studies. *Anesthesiology.* 2005;103:1238-1245.
5. Akata T, Murakami J, Yoshinaga A. Life-threatening haemorrhage following obturator artery injury during transurethral bladder surgery: a sequel of an unsuccessful obturator nerve block. *Acta Anaesthesiol Scand.* 1999;43:784-788.
6. Woodburne RT. The accessory obturator nerve and the innervation of the pectineus muscle. *Anat Rec.* 1960;136:367-369.

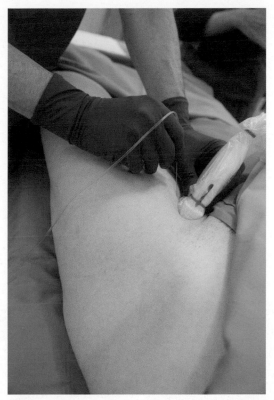

Figure 42-1. External photograph showing the approach to obturator nerve block in the medial thigh. An out-of-plane approach is shown.

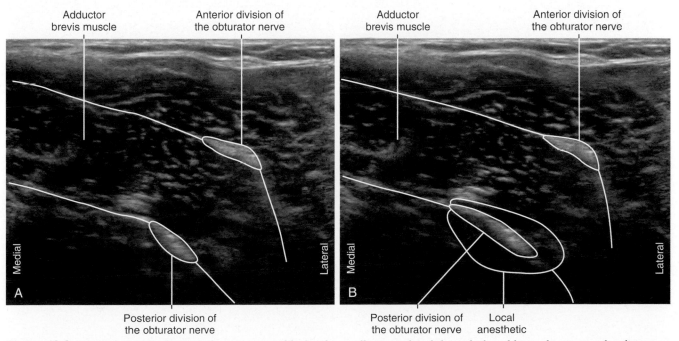

Figure 42-2. Image sequence showing obturator nerve block. The needle tip is placed through the adductor brevis muscle adjacent to the posterior division of the obturator nerve in an out-of-plane approach (**A**). After injection, local anesthetic is distributed around the posterior division (**B**). In this example, the posterior division is well visualized.

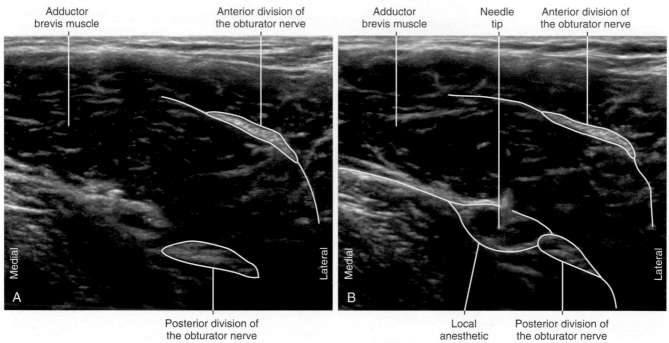

Figure 42-3. Image sequence showing obturator nerve block. The needle tip is placed through the adductor brevis muscle adjacent to the posterior division of the obturator nerve in an out-of-plane approach (**A**). After injection, local anesthetic is distributed around the posterior division (**B**). In this example, the anterior division is well visualized.

CHAPTER 43

SCIATIC NERVE BLOCK

Proximal sciatic nerve block is a versatile regional anesthetic for lower extremity surgery. It is usually combined with femoral nerve block for more complete anesthesia of the leg. The sciatic nerve (L4 to S3) is the largest nerve in the body, with a transverse diameter of more than 17 mm on ultrasound scans.[1] However, despite its large size, the sciatic nerve can be difficult to visualize in the gluteal region and proximal thigh. Sonographic features of the regional anatomy are essential to identifying the nerve.

Suggested Technique

The subgluteal region has a "bright triangle" consisting of the hyperechoic sciatic nerve and adjacent tendons of the semitendinosus-biceps and semimembranosus. These proximal tendons can appear similar to the sciatic nerve. The sciatic nerve is always lateral to these ischiocrural tendons. The long head of the biceps femoris overlies the short head. The semimembranosus is characterized by a large, flat proximal aponeurosis. The semitendinosus has a more round proximal tendon. Short-axis view with sliding of the transducer is better than long-axis view to confirm nerve identity and distinguish it from the adjacent tendons.

Prone position allows the most stable access for proximal sciatic nerve block. In-plane technique from the lateral side of the leg is a relatively easy approach to proximal sciatic block. If prone positioning is difficult, lateral approach also is possible for this block. A broad linear probe (5-cm footprint or larger) is best to provide a large field of view for this block because working room is not limited in this region.

Anatomic variation of the sciatic nerve in the subgluteal region primarily consists of identification of separate contributions from the common peroneal and tibial nerves.[2,3] This indicates proximal division of the sciatic nerve by the piriformis muscle. If the anomaly is correctly identified, multiple-injection technique guided by ultrasound provides complete sciatic block.

The sciatic nerve lies about halfway between the greater trochanter (lateral) and the ischial tuberosity (medial). These bony reference points are useful proximal landmarks for sciatic block in the gluteal region.[4] In some patients, the inferior gluteal artery can be identified on the medial side of the proximal sciatic nerve.

Clinical Pearls

- A number of patient positions can be used to approach proximal sciatic nerve block. Prone position is favored because of the stable imaging for in-plane technique from the lateral aspect of the thigh. Another relatively easy alternative is the lateral position with a hip bump to provide stability.
- When an accompanying artery is identified on the lateral side of the sciatic nerve, place the needle tip in the connective tissue between the nerve and the artery. This may require puncturing the connective tissue with the block needle and slowly injecting as the needle is withdrawn to identify the correct layer surrounding the nerve.
- The fascia surrounding the sciatic nerve in the subgluteal region is thick. This emphasizes the importance of correct needle tip positioning and local anesthetic distribution.

References

1. Heinemeyer O, Reimers CD. Ultrasound of radial, ulnar, median, and sciatic nerves in healthy subjects and patients with hereditary motor and sensory neuropathies. *Ultrasound Med Biol*. 1999;25:481-485.
2. Benzon HT, Katz JA, Benzon HA, Iqbal MS. Piriformis syndrome: anatomic considerations, a new injection technique, and a review of the literature. *Anesthesiology*. 2003;98:1442-1448.
3. Pokorny D, Jahoda D, Veigl D, et al. Topographic variations of the relationship of the sciatic nerve and the piriformis muscle and its relevance to palsy after total hip arthroplasty. *Surg Radiol Anat*. 2006;28:88-91.
4. Chan VW, Nova H, Abbas S, et al. Ultrasound examination and localization of the sciatic nerve: a volunteer study. *Anesthesiology*. 2006;104:309-314.

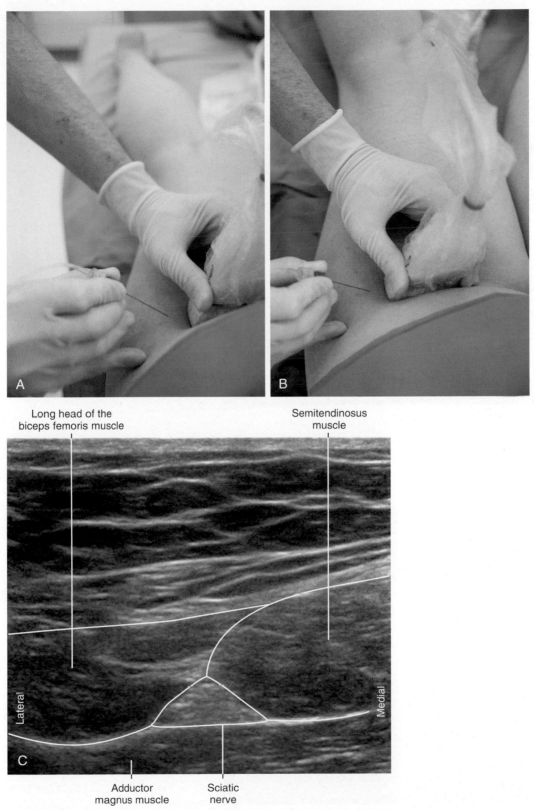

Long head of the
biceps femoris muscle

Semitendinosus
muscle

Lateral

Medial

Adductor
magnus muscle

Sciatic
nerve

Figure 43-1. External photograph showing the approach to sciatic nerve block in the subgluteal region. An in-plane approach from the lateral aspect of the thigh is shown (**A** and **B**). The corresponding sonogram with the sciatic nerve in transverse view is shown (**C**). The subgluteal sciatic nerve often has a triangular shape defined by the following three borders: the long head of the biceps femoris (posterolateral), the semi-tendinosus (posteromedial), and the adductor magnus (anterior). Sciatic nerve block usually targets the lateral corner of the nerve.

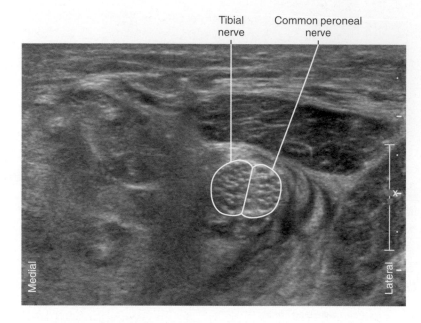

Figure 43-2. Echotexture of the sciatic nerve. In some subjects, the tibial and common peroneal components can be visualized within the sciatic nerve.

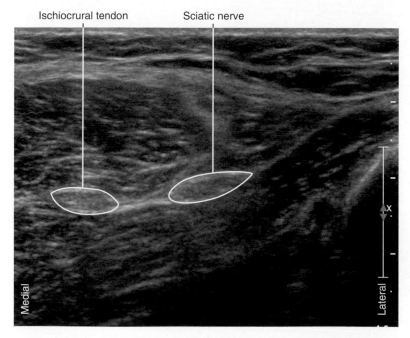

Figure 43-3. Depending on the location of imaging, the ischiocrural tendons can appear similar to the sciatic nerve on ultrasound scans. The sciatic nerve always lies lateral to these tendons.

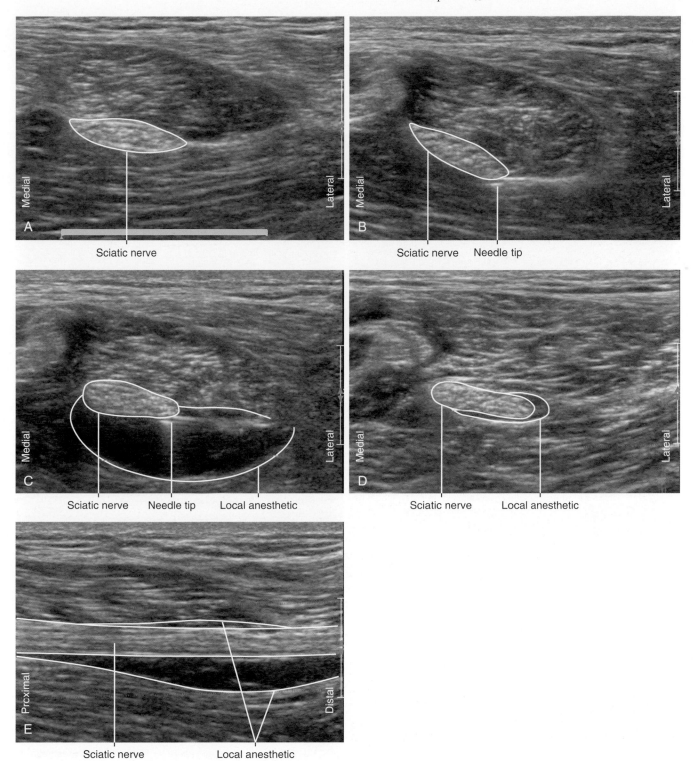

Figure 43-4. Image sequence showing sciatic nerve block in the subgluteal region. A short-axis view of the sciatic nerve is shown before needle placement (**A**). An in-plane approach from the lateral aspect of the thigh is demonstrated where the needle tip is placed at the lateral corner of the nerve (**B**) with injection of local anesthetic (**C**). After injection, local anesthetic is distributed around the sciatic nerve (**D**) and tracks along the nerve (**E**). Note that the fascia that surrounds the sciatic nerve in the subgluteal region is thick, and careful assessment of the local anesthetic distribution is necessary if surgical anesthesia is desired.

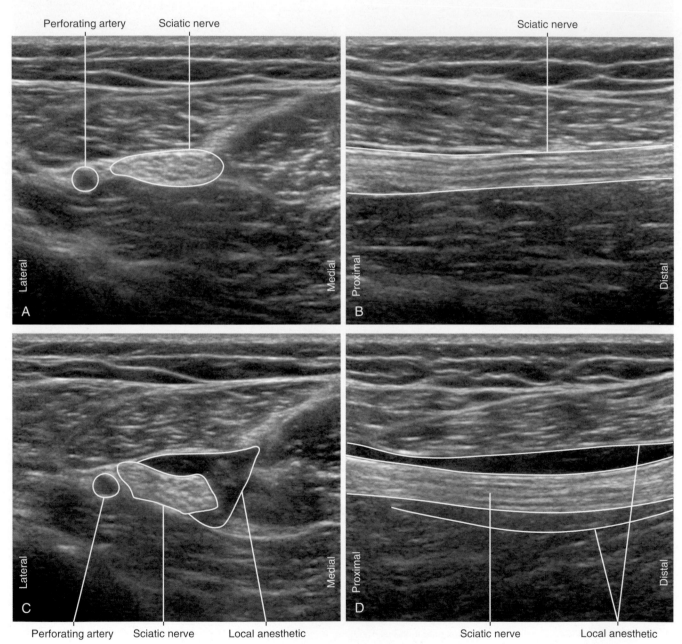

Figure 43-5. Sciatic nerve local anesthetic distributions. Short-axis (**A**) and long-axis (**B**) views of the sciatic nerve at the start of injection of local anesthetic. Short-axis (**C**) and long-axis (**D**) views of the sciatic nerve after completion of the injection of local anesthetic.

CHAPTER 44

POPLITEAL BLOCK

Popliteal sciatic nerve blocks are versatile regional anesthetics that provide surgical anesthesia of the foot and ankle. These blocks are often combined with saphenous or femoral nerve blocks for complete anesthesia of the distal leg. The idea behind popliteal blocks is to perform the procedure near where the sciatic nerve divides into its tibial and common peroneal components. The only anatomic structure that bifurcates in the popliteal fossa is the sciatic nerve.

The tibial nerve visibility is best near the knee crease because of the relatively small extremity size. In that location, the typical anatomy is popliteal artery, popliteal vein, and tibial nerve (listed from deep to superficial within a parasagittal plane). The tibial nerve is about twice the size of the common peroneal nerve in terms of cross-sectional area.[1] The tibial nerve has a straight course near the middle of the lower extremity, whereas the common peroneal nerve has a more oblique (lateral) course.

The common peroneal nerve will travel distally with the conjoint tendon of the biceps femoris. The common peroneal nerve is posterior to the conjoint tendon of the biceps femoris near the knee crease. With the foot in neutral position, the common peroneal nerve usually lies slightly closer to the posterior surface of the leg than the tibial nerve.[2] Because it is smaller and has fewer fascicles, the common peroneal nerve is more difficult to identify than the tibial nerve.[3]

Suggested Technique

Elevation of the leg and some internal rotation will allow imaging of the popliteal fossa from the posterior surface.[4] A broad linear transducer (35-50 mm footprint, 10 MHz) is used for adult patients. The choice of block needle (7-9 cm, 20-22 gauge) is not critical.

Popliteal block is usually performed just distal to the sciatic nerve bifurcation in the popliteal fossa for several reasons. First, the nerves are close to the posterior skin surface. This makes nerve imaging and positioning the needle tip easier. Second, the needle can be aimed at the connective tissue space between the tibial and common peroneal nerves (rather than directly aimed at the sciatic nerve).[5] The block is performed where the tibial and common peroneal nerves are about one needle-width apart (about 1 mm). Third, there is a large amount of nerve surface area available for diffusion of local anesthetic to promote clinical block characteristics. The point of sonographic unity is closer to the knee crease than anatomic dissections would suggest because the tibial and common peroneal nerves run next to each other for some distance before visibly separating. The only disadvantage to this more distal popliteal block is that the popliteal vessels are closer to the nerves.

The needle bevel should face toward the transducer for optimal needle tip visibility (bevel down). Because the common peroneal nerve is slightly closer to the posterior surface than the tibial nerve, it is best to approach the gap between the two nerves from the femur side (i.e., a slight posterior inclination of the block needle with lateral approach).

Recent studies have suggested a limited ability of ultrasound to correctly assess circumferential distribution of local anesthetic around peripheral nerves. The reported predictive value of the "doughnut" sign is only about 90% for sciatic nerve blocks.[6] One major advantage to sciatic nerve block in the popliteal fossa is that it allows sliding assessment of the longitudinal distribution along the nerve branches (i.e., local anesthetic should not only surround the nerve but also track along the nerves).

The onset of blockade of the common peroneal nerve is usually faster than for the tibial nerve, which may reflect the smaller size of the common peroneal nerve.[7]

Clinical Pearls

- Leg elevation and internal rotation help ultrasound-guided blocks in supine position.
- The posterior cutaneous nerve of the thigh plays little role in thigh tourniquet tolerance.
- The only major branches of the sciatic nerve in the thigh are the tibial and common peroneal nerves. The connective tissue between these two nerves is the target for the block needle tip.
- Movement of the foot induces characteristic nerve motion in the popliteal fossa that can improve nerve conspicuity (the "seesaw" sign).[2]
- A hip bump will help rotate the leg into favorable position for popliteal block.
- Slight reverse Trendelenburg position will level the posterior surface of the leg for imaging.
- Ultrasound guidance is particularly useful for locating the bifurcation of the sciatic nerve into the tibial and common peroneal nerves. Rare cases of proximal division of the sciatic nerve (16 cm proximal to the knee crease) have been revealed with ultrasound imaging.[8]

References

1. Heinemeyer O, Reimers CD. Ultrasound of radial, ulnar, median, and sciatic nerves in healthy subjects and patients with hereditary motor and sensory neuropathies. *Ultrasound Med Biol.* 1999;25:481-485.
2. Schafhalter-Zoppoth I, Younger SJ, Collins AB, Gray AT. The "seesaw" sign: improved sonographic identification of the sciatic nerve. *Anesthesiology.* 2004;101:808-809.
3. Peeters EY, Nieboer KH, Osteaux MM. Sonography of the normal ulnar nerve at Guyon's canal and of the common peroneal nerve dorsal to the fibular head. *J Clin Ultrasound.* 2004;32:375-380.
4. Gray AT, Huczko EL, Schafhalter-Zoppoth I. Lateral popliteal nerve block with ultrasound guidance. *Reg Anesth Pain Med.* 2004;29:507-509.
5. Vloka JD, Hadžić A, Lesser JB, et al. A common epineural sheath for the nerves in the popliteal fossa and its possible implications for sciatic nerve block. *Anesth Analg.* 1997;84:387-390.
6. Perlas A, Brull R, Chan VW, et al. Ultrasound guidance improves the success of sciatic nerve block at the popliteal fossa. *Reg Anesth Pain Med.* 2008;33:259-265.
7. Paqueron X, Bouaziz H, Macalou D, et al. The lateral approach to the sciatic nerve at the popliteal fossa: one or two injections? *Anesth Analg.* 1999;89:1221-1225.
8. Clendenen SR, York JE, Wang RD, Greengrass RA. Three-dimensional ultrasound-assisted popliteal catheter placement revealing aberrant anatomy: implications for block failure. *Acta Anaesthesiol Scand.* 2008;52:1429-1431.

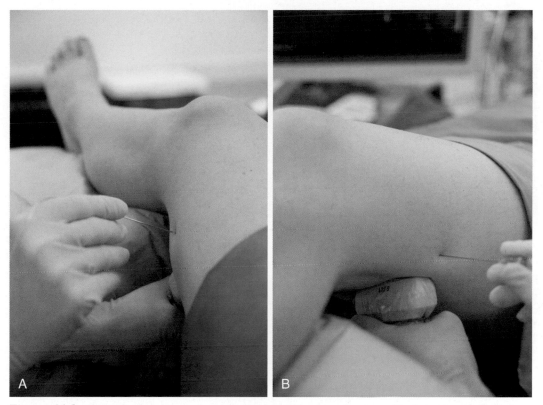

Figure 44-1. External photograph showing the approach to sciatic nerve block in the popliteal fossa (**A** and **B**). An in-plane approach from the lateral aspect of the thigh is shown. The patient is supine with the leg elevated to allow access for the transducer from the posterior aspect of the leg. Internal rotation of the leg also helps ultrasound-guided blocks in supine position.

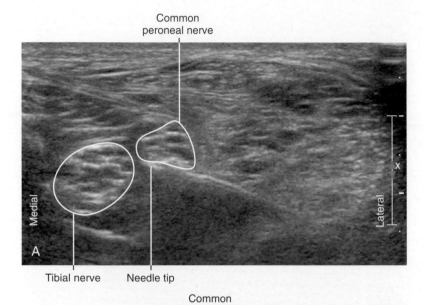

Common
peroneal nerve

Tibial nerve   Needle tip

Common
peroneal nerve

Tibial nerve   Needle tip   Local anesthetic

Figure 44-2. Image sequence showing popliteal block. An in-plane approach is demonstrated whereby the needle tip is placed between the common peroneal and tibial nerves (**A**). The block needle is then advanced until tent and recoil of the adjoining connective tissue is observed. After injection, local anesthetic is distributed around both nerves (**B**).

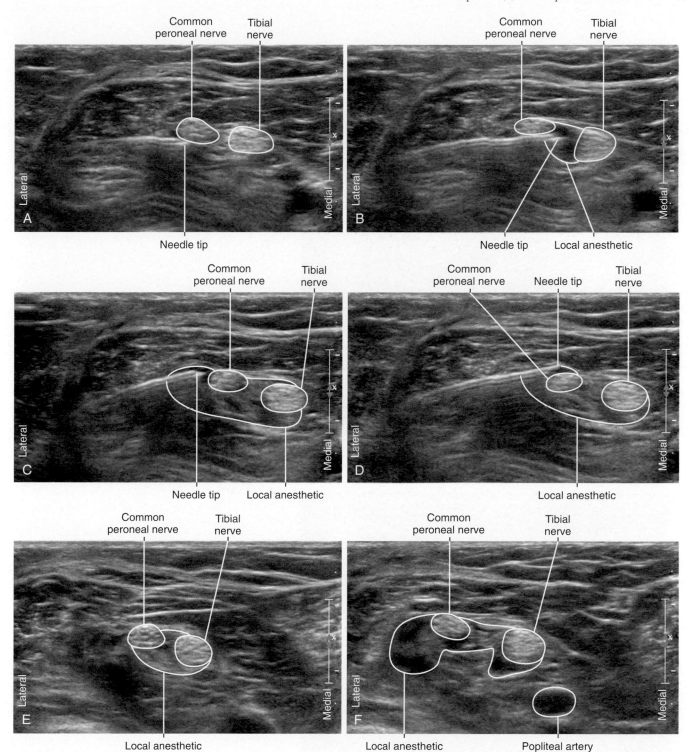

Figure 44-3. Image sequence showing popliteal block. An in-plane approach is demonstrated in which the needle tip is placed between the common peroneal and tibial nerves (**A**). After injection, local anesthetic is distributed around both nerves (**B**). Additional local anesthetic is deposited around the common peroneal nerve by rotating the bevel of the block needle (**C** and **D**). Sliding along the nerves demonstrates the local anesthetic distribution to both nerves (**E** and **F**).

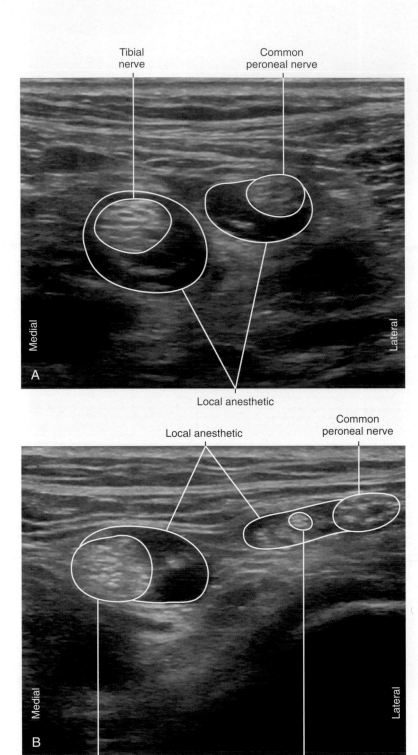

Tibial
nerve

Common
peroneal nerve

Medial

Lateral

A

Local anesthetic

Local anesthetic

Common
peroneal nerve

Medial

Lateral

B

Tibial nerve

Contribution to
sural nerve

Figure 44-4. Local anesthetic distribution after popliteal block. By sliding the transducer along the known course of the nerves, local anesthetic is seen to distribute to both the common peroneal and tibial nerves (**A**). By sliding the transducer even more distally, a third nerve within local anesthetic is now identified (**B**). This nerve is the common peroneal contribution to the sural nerve and the lateral cutaneous nerve of the leg. When multiple rings of local anesthetic are identified that track along nerve branches, the resultant block is unequivocal.

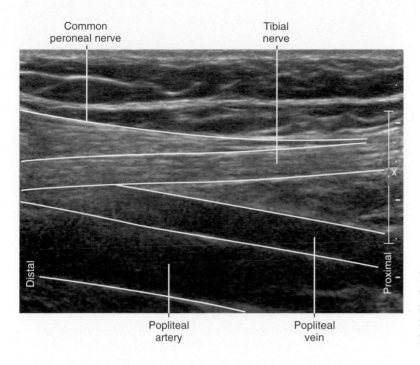

Common
peroneal nerve

Tibial
nerve

Distal

Proximal

Popliteal
artery

Popliteal
vein

Figure 44-5. Long-axis view of the popliteal fossa. In this sonogram, the usual courses of the common peroneal nerve, tibial nerve, popliteal vein, and popliteal artery are illustrated in one parasagittal plane of imaging (listed from posterior to anterior).

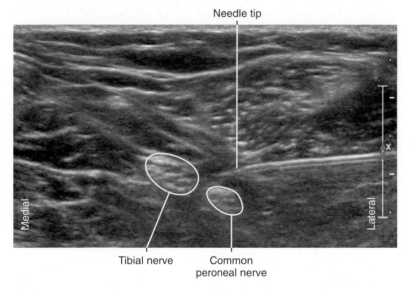

Needle tip

Medial

Lateral

Tibial nerve

Common
peroneal nerve

Figure 44-6. Nerve position for popliteal block. In most cases, the common peroneal nerve lies closer to the posterior surface of the thigh than does the tibial nerve. However, the location of these nerves depends on foot position, and in some cases, the tibial nerve will lie closer to the posterior surface (as shown here).

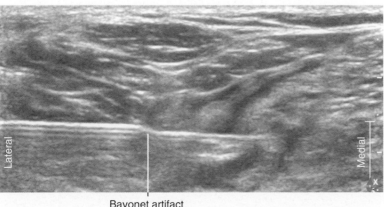

Lateral

Medial

Bayonet artifact

Figure 44-7. Bayonet artifact during popliteal block. Because the angle of approach is near parallel to the active face of the transducer, bayonet artifacts can be observed during popliteal blocks. This speed-of-sound artifact causes apparent bending of the needle (although no actual mechanical bending of the needle exists).

CHAPTER 45

ANKLE BLOCK

Ankle block is a useful regional anesthetic technique for foot surgery, especially in the ambulatory setting.[1] Additionally, ankle block provides excellent postoperative analgesia, which is important because foot surgeries often involve several osteotomies that cause moderate to severe postoperative pain, which is difficult to manage with standard oral analgesic regimens.

The foot is innervated by five nerves: four are terminal branches of the sciatic nerve, and one is the terminal branch of the femoral nerve. Many of the nerves of the foot can be directly imaged with ultrasound. This approach is more targeted than traditional ankle blocks. Using ultrasound guidance, it may be possible to improve patient comfort during the procedure and produce more complete blocks. In addition, more proximal blocks of the foot may be indicated when edema or infection is present. In contrast to blocks of the sciatic nerve in the popliteal fossa, ankle blocks do not produce foot drop, and therefore patient disposition is potentially facilitated.

Reference

1. Monkowski DP, Egidi HR. Ankle block. *Tech Reg Anesth Pain Manag.* 2006;10:183-188.

46

DEEP PERONEAL
NERVE BLOCK

The deep peroneal nerve is a small branch of the common peroneal nerve. The deep peroneal nerve innervates the web space between the first and second toes. The nerve crosses over the anterior tibial artery from medial to lateral just proximal to the ankle joint near the surface of the distal tibia. The deep peroneal nerve often appears as a homogeneous hypoechoic structure surrounded by hyperechoic fat without fascicular echotexture.

Suggested Technique

The deep peroneal nerve and anterior tibial artery lie between the surface of the tibia and the extensor hallucis longus muscle. Because of its superficial location and proximity to bone, the anterior tibial artery is easily compressed by the transducer over the dorsum of the foot and ankle. Light touch with the transducer is necessary to image the anterior tibial artery. By sliding the transducer back and forth from proximal to distal, the crossing of the deep peroneal nerve over the anterior tibial artery can be identified. Both in-plane and out-of-plane approaches are useful for this block.

The deep peroneal nerve is difficult to image in the proximal leg.[1] This probably relates to the course of the nerve and its division into a large number of motor branches.[2]

Clinical Pearls

- Because the deep peroneal nerve is small, it is difficult to visualize where it branches off from the common peroneal nerve in the proximal leg.
- The point at which the deep peroneal nerve crosses over the anterior tibial artery is typically proximal to the ankle joint where the artery lies on the surface of the tibia.
- The deep peroneal nerve divides into medial and lateral branches. These branches lie on their respective sides of the anterior tibial artery.
- The deep peroneal nerve can be blocked by peeling off the nerve from the anterior tibial artery where it lies in the 12-o'clock position with respect to the artery (at the crossing point). A more proximal approach is to lift up the nerve from the lateral side of the artery before it crosses over. Blocking the deep peroneal nerve on the medial side of the artery is not recommended because the nerve may have already branched into medial and lateral components.

References

1. Beekman R, Visser LH. High-resolution sonography of the peripheral nervous system: a review of the literature. *Eur J Neurol.* 2004;11:305-314.
2. Aigner F, Longato S, Gardetto A, et al. Anatomic survey of the common fibular nerve and its branching pattern with regard to the intermuscular septa of the leg. *Clin Anat.* 2004;17:503-512.

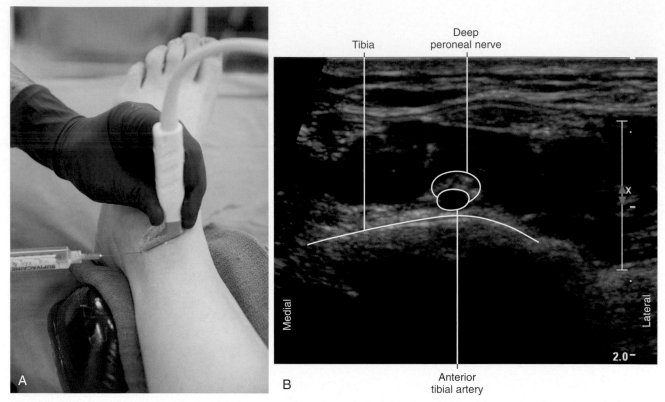

Figure 46-1. External photograph showing the approach to deep peroneal block in the distal leg. An in-plane approach from the lateral aspect of the leg is shown (**A**). The corresponding sonogram is shown before needle placement (**B**). The deep peroneal nerve crosses over the surface of the anterior tibial artery proximal to the ankle joint.

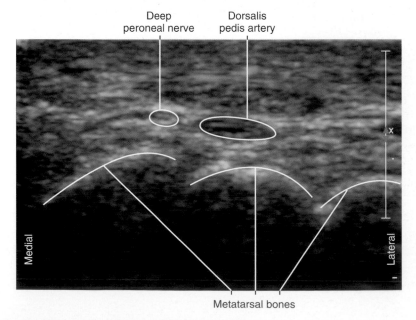

Figure 46-2. Short-axis view of the deep peroneal nerve over the dorsum of the foot. In this more distal location, the metatarsal bones lie under the nerve. This location is too distal for complete block.

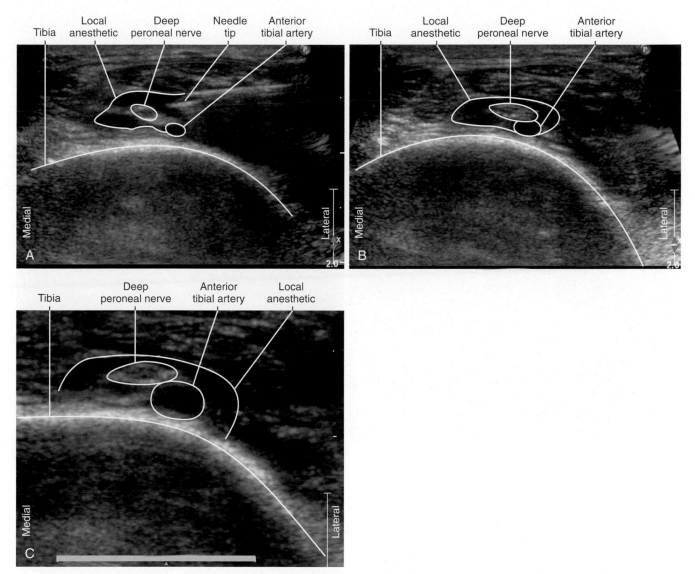

Figure 46-3. Image sequence showing deep peroneal nerve block in the distal leg. At this location, the deep peroneal nerve lies over the anterior tibial artery. An in-plane approach is demonstrated in which the needle tip is placed adjacent to the anterior tibial artery and the deep peroneal nerve with the nerve in the 12-o'clock position (**A**). After injection, local anesthetic is distributed around the deep peroneal nerve and begins to separate the nerve from the artery (**B**), also shown at higher magnification (**C**).

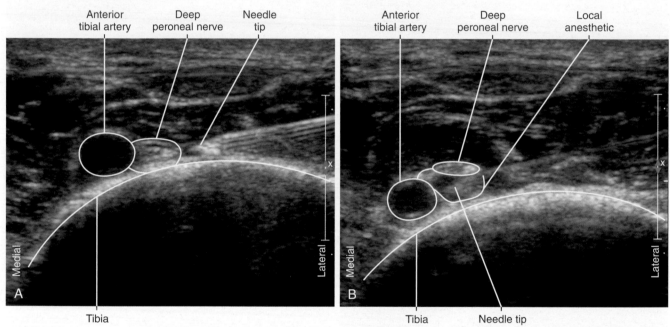

Figure 46-4. Image sequence showing deep peroneal nerve block in the distal leg. At this location, the deep peroneal nerve lies on the side of the anterior tibial artery. An in-plane approach is demonstrated in which the needle tip is placed under the deep peroneal nerve (**A**). After injection, the local anesthetic lifts the nerve from the surface of the bone (**B**).

SUPERFICIAL PERONEAL NERVE BLOCK

The superficial peroneal nerve is a branch of the common peroneal nerve that emerges from the neck of the fibula between the extensor digitorum longus and peroneal muscles to enter the subcutaneous tissue of the lateral leg. When emerging from the fibular neck, the superficial peroneal nerve most commonly lies in the lateral compartment of the leg. The superficial peroneal nerve travels up along the anterior intermuscular septum to pierce the fascia lata at the juncture of the middle and lower thirds of the leg. The nerve divides into its medial and lateral branches once in the subcutaneous tissue.

Superficial peroneal nerve block in the leg can be useful when edema or infection contraindicates more distal ankle block. Proximal ultrasound-guided superficial peroneal nerve block (along with sural block) can provide surgical anesthesia for hardware removal from the lateral ankle in weight-bearing patients. In addition, ultrasound-guided superficial block in the leg is less painful than subcutaneous infiltration across the dorsum of the foot for more distal block.

Suggested Technique

The superficial peroneal nerve can be difficult to image within the subcutaneous tissue of the distal lateral leg. By sliding the transducer along the known course of the nerve, the nerve can be identified as it emerges from the muscular compartment. An in-plane approach from the posterolateral side of the leg can then be used for needle tip placement adjacent to the nerve.

More proximally, the peroneal nerves are best imaged in the prone position with the knee flexed using a pillow under the ankle.[1,2] Alternatively, the leg can be elevated and internally rotated with the patient in supine position. When scanning from distal to proximal, the superficial peroneal nerve tracks along the fascia between the anterior and lateral compartments of the leg (like going down a ski jump), until it meets the acute edge of the bone of the fibula. The anterior border of the fibula is formed by the insertion of the anterior intermuscular septum. Because the nerve tracks along the anterior intermuscular septum, the anterior border of the fibula will point toward the superficial peroneal nerve.

Because the superficial peroneal nerve most often lies in the lateral compartment side of the intermuscular septum,[3] it is important for the block needle tip to puncture the septum when approaching from the anterior side. The block needle tip crosses the anterior intermuscular septum under the nerve, with injection of local anesthetic as the needle is pulled back. If the nerve is blocked close to the surface of the fascia lata, its deeper motor branches to the peroneus longus and peroneus brevis can be spared.

Clinical Pearls

- Begin by scanning anterior and proximal to the lateral malleolus with the probe perpendicular to the known course of the superficial peroneal nerve.
- The superficial peroneal nerve emerges in the groove between the extensor digitorum longus and peroneal muscles.
- As a rule, the more proximal the branches of the superficial peroneal nerve pierce the fascia lata, the more likely it is that their course will stay parallel with the fibula.[4,5]
- When the superficial peroneal nerve is divided by the intermuscular septum it continues distally as the medial and intermediate dorsal cutaneous nerves of the foot.
- When two adjacent nerves are identified within the field of view, confirm that they join proximally.
- The diameters of the superficial peroneal nerve and its branches are approximately 3 and 2 mm, respectively.[6]
- Conditions that contraindicate ankle block (e.g., edema and infection) are not common in outpatients. Popliteal blocks are much more commonly used than more distal blocks in these settings because patient disposition is not an issue.

References

1. Peer S, Kovacs P, Harpf C, Bodner G. High-resolution sonography of lower extremity peripheral nerves: anatomic correlation and spectrum of disease. *J Ultrasound Med.* 2002;21:315-322.
2. Gruber H, Peer S, Meirer R, Bodner G. Peroneal nerve palsy associated with knee luxation: evaluation by sonography. Initial experiences. *AJR Am J Roentgenol.* 2005;185:1119-1125.
3. Ducic I, Dellon AL, Graw KS. The clinical importance of variations in the surgical anatomy of the superficial peroneal nerve in the mid-third of the lateral leg. *Ann Plast Surg.* 2006;56:635-638.
4. Saito A, Kikuchi S. Anatomic relations between ankle arthroscopic portal sites and the superficial peroneal and saphenous nerves. *Foot Ankle Int.* 1998;19:748-752.
5. Solomon LB, Ferris L, Tedman R, Henneberg M. Surgical anatomy of the sural and superficial fibular nerves with an emphasis on the approach to the lateral malleolus. *J Anat.* 2001;199:717-723.
6. Sayli U, Tekdemyr Y, Çubuk HE, et al. The course of the superficial peroneal nerve: an anatomical cadaver study. *Foot Ankle Surg.* 1998;4:63-69.

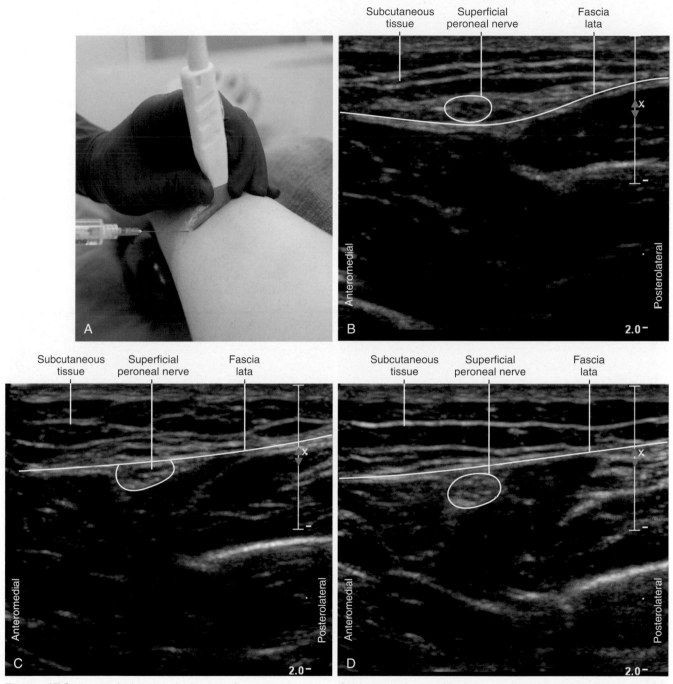

Figure 47-1. External photograph showing the approach to superficial peroneal nerve block in the distal leg. An in-plane approach from the posterolateral aspect of the leg is shown (**A**). The corresponding sonogram shows the nerve within the subcutaneous tissue of the lateral leg (**B**). More proximal sonograms show the nerve emerging from the muscular compartment (**C** and **D**).

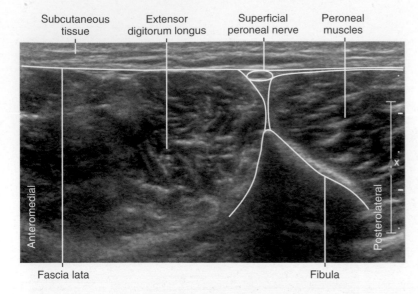

Figure 47-2. The superficial peroneal nerve arises from the common peroneal nerve near the neck of the fibula in the proximal leg. The edge of the bone is sharp and points to the superficial peroneal nerve because the nerve emerges within or adjacent to the intermuscular septum.

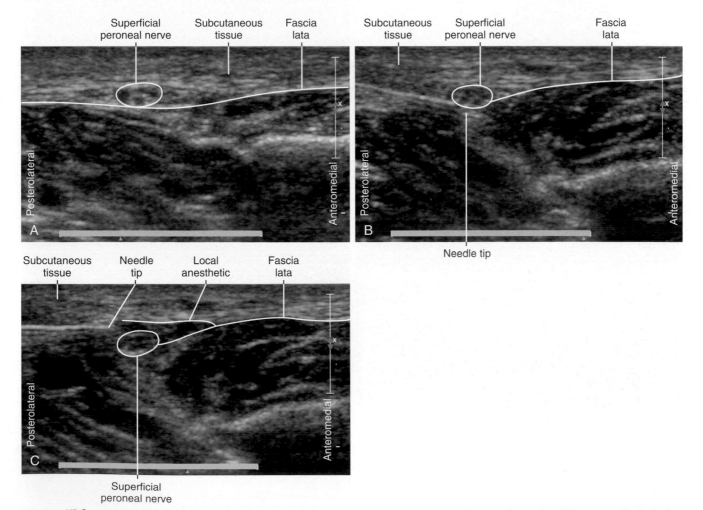

Figure 47-3. Image sequence showing superficial peroneal nerve block in the distal leg. The superficial peroneal nerve is shown before needle placement (**A**). An in-plane approach is demonstrated where the needle tip is placed under the nerve (**B**). After injection, local anesthetic is distributed around the superficial peroneal nerve (**C**).

CHAPTER 48

SURAL NERVE BLOCK

The sural nerve forms from branches of the tibial (medial) and common peroneal (lateral) components of the sciatic nerve. Although the sural usually receives both contributions, anatomic variation is common.

The sural nerve lies adjacent to the small saphenous vein within the subcutaneous tissue of the lateral leg. The sural nerve provides sensory innervation to the lateral foot.[1] Because it is a sensory nerve, the sural nerve is sometimes used for biopsy or harvest. Although subcutaneous infiltration is an effective means of blocking the distal sural nerve, more proximal block may be indicated in patients with infection or edema of the foot.

Suggested Technique

Because of its small size, the sural nerve can be difficult to image.[2] The sural nerve can be blocked proximal to the lateral malleolus by applying a calf tourniquet to help identify the small saphenous vein. In this location, the sural nerve lies adjacent to the vein within the subcutaneous tissue of the leg. An in-plane approach can be used to distribute local anesthetic around the sural nerve.

A sural contribution from the tibial nerve can often be imaged between the medial and lateral heads of the gastrocnemius muscle. This contribution emerges between these muscles to pierce the fascia lata and join the lesser saphenous vein and the common peroneal nerve contribution within the subcutaneous tissue of the lateral aspect of the lower leg.[3] The sural nerve can be blocked with an in-plane approach from the lateral aspect of the leg with the patient in supine position and the leg elevated. Although prone position is optimal for sural nerve imaging, the former approach is more practical and useful in most patients.

Clinical Pearls

- The sural nerve emerges between the medial and lateral heads of the gastrocnemius to enter the subcutaneous tissue of the calf adjacent to the small saphenous vein.
- The sural nerve and small saphenous vein pass posterior to the lateral malleolus.
- Because the sural nerve lies in subcutaneous tissue in this location, it will not be mistaken for a nearby tendon.

References

1. Solomon LB, Ferris L, Tedman R, Henneberg M. Surgical anatomy of the sural and superficial fibular nerves with an emphasis on the approach to the lateral malleolus. *J Anat.* 2001;199:717-723.
2. Simonetti S, Bianchi S, Martinoli C. Neurophysiological and ultrasound findings in sural nerve lesions following stripping of the small saphenous vein. *Muscle Nerve.* 1999;22:1724-1726.
3. Coert JH, Dellon AL. Clinical implications of the surgical anatomy of the sural nerve. *Plast Reconstr Surg.* 1994;94:850-855.

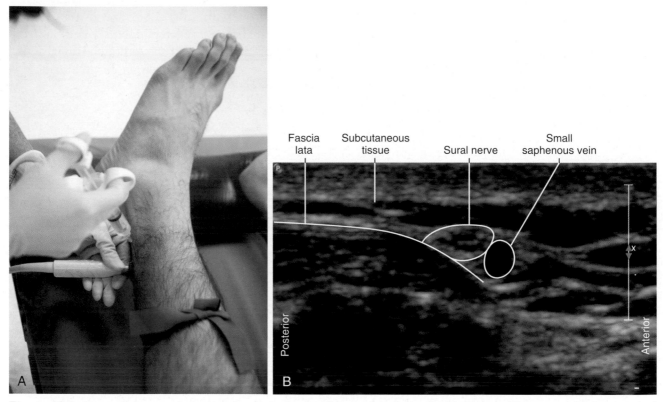

Figure 48-1. External photograph showing the approach to sural nerve block in the distal leg (**A**). A calf tourniquet has been applied to improve the visibility of the small saphenous vein behind the lateral malleolus. The corresponding sonogram is shown (**B**). The sural nerve is adjacent to the small saphenous vein within the subcutaneous tissue of the posterolateral leg. The nerve and vein are viewed in short axis.

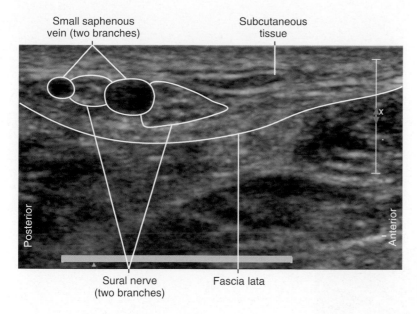

Figure 48-2. Short-axis view of the sural nerve in the distal leg. In some patients, the sural nerve and adjacent small saphenous vein are divided.

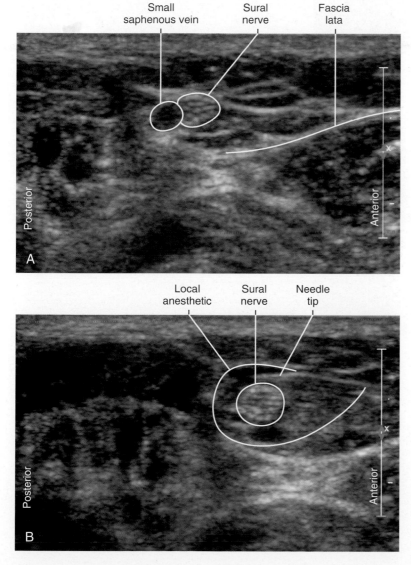

Figure 48-3. Image sequence showing sural nerve block in the distal leg. Before injection, the sural nerve is identified adjacent to the small saphenous vein (**A**). An in-plane approach is demonstrated where the needle tip is placed adjacent to the sural nerve within the subcutaneous tissue of the leg (**B**). Local anesthetic surrounds the sural nerve and compresses the small saphenous vein.

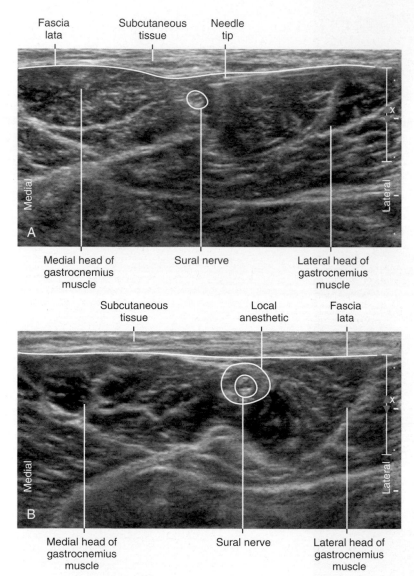

Fascia lata · **Subcutaneous tissue** · **Needle tip**

Medial

Lateral

A

Medial head of gastrocnemius muscle · **Sural nerve** · **Lateral head of gastrocnemius muscle**

Subcutaneous tissue · **Local anesthetic** · **Fascia lata**

Medial

Lateral

B

Medial head of gastrocnemius muscle · **Sural nerve** · **Lateral head of gastrocnemius muscle**

Figure 48-4. Proximal sural nerve block. The sural nerve also can be blocked in the posterior calf where it emerges between the medial and lateral heads of the gastrocnemius muscle into the subcutaneous tissue of the leg (**A** and **B**).

TIBIAL NERVE BLOCK

The tibial nerve is the largest branch of the sciatic nerve and the largest nerve for the ankle block. It provides sensory innervation to the heel and to the sole of the foot. The tibial nerve divides into the medial calcaneal, medial plantar, and lateral plantar branches near the ankle.[1] In some subjects, the takeoff of the medial calcaneal branch from the tibial nerve can be imaged above the ankle joint.

The order of anatomic structures from anterior to posterior at the medial malleolus is: Tom, Dick, AVN, Harry (**t**ibialis posterior tendon, flexor **d**igitorum longus tendon, posterior tibial **a**rtery and **v**eins, tibial **n**erve, flexor **h**allucis longus tendon). Therefore, the tibial nerve lies on the heel side of the posterior tibial artery. The posterior tibial artery is often accompanied by two flanking veins. This neurovascular bundle, consisting of one artery and two veins, can have a Mickey Mouse ears appearance if light touch with the transducer is applied (similar to the appearance of the brachial artery and veins in the arm).

Edema or infection often makes routine ankle block ineffective or contraindicated.[2,3] However, tibial nerve imaging can be difficult in some surgical patients with peripheral vascular disease because vascular landmarks of the nerve are not present. Tibial nerve block in the leg avoids the foot drop that occurs with more proximal popliteal block of the sciatic nerve. This can be an advantage for ambulatory surgery patients.

Suggested Technique

The tibial nerve can be approached in-plane from the anterior (tibial) side in supine position with the leg externally rotated using a short-axis view of the neurovascular bundle. The best point of tibial nerve imaging in the leg is usually halfway between the medial malleolus and the bulk of the gastrocnemius-soleus muscle complex in the calf. Place the block needle tip between the posterior tibial artery and the tibial nerve so as to enter the neurovascular compartment. With this approach, the saphenous vein can be close to the needle path near the skin surface.

Clinical Pearls

- The ideal needle path is between the posterior tibial artery and the tibial nerve, so that the injection separates the two structures.
- Tibial nerve block with ultrasound can be used for outpatient heel surgery to avoid foot drop that occurs with more proximal popliteal block of the sciatic nerve.
- The medial calcaneal branch of the tibial nerve can sometimes be imaged, particularly after tibial nerve block in the leg.
- Be careful with long-axis assessments of local anesthetic distribution along peripheral nerves that lie close to arteries (e.g., the tibial nerve). Partial line-ups on the adjacent artery can appear similar to distributed fluid.
- The central aponeurosis of the tibialis posterior muscle lies deep to the tibial nerve in the leg. These two structures can have similar ultrasound appearance.
- Tibial nerve block also can be approached from the Achilles tendon side (with leg slightly elevated and flexed).

References

1. Bareither DJ, Genau JM, Massaro JC. Variation in the division of the tibial nerve: application to nerve blocks. *J Foot Surg.* 1990;29:581-583.
2. Larrabure P, Pandin P, Vancutsem N, Vandesteene A. Tibial nerve block: evaluation of a novel midleg approach in 241 patients. *Can J Anaesth.* 2005;52:276-280.
3. Soares LG, Brull R, Chan VW. Teaching an old block a new trick: ultrasound-guided posterior tibial nerve block. *Acta Anaesthesiol Scand.* 2008;52:446-447.

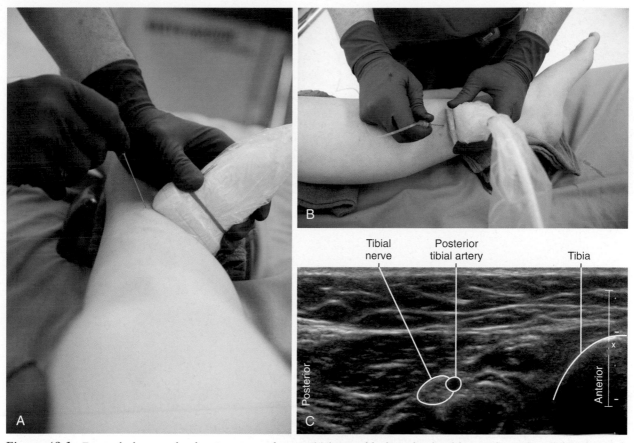

Figure 49-1. External photographs showing approaches to tibial nerve block in the distal leg. Both in-plane (**A**) and out-of-plane (**B**) approaches are shown. The corresponding ultrasound scan is shown (**C**). This location is proximal to where the tibial nerve divides into its medial plantar, lateral plantar, and medial calcaneal branches.

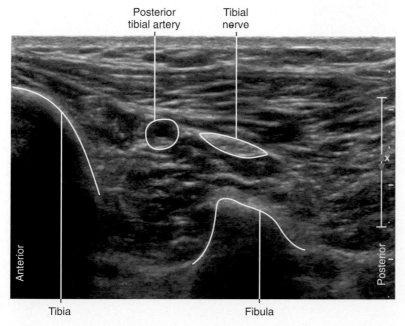

Figure 49-2. Short-axis view of the tibial nerve in the distal leg. With a broad and deep view, both the tibia and fibula can be imaged deep to the nerve.

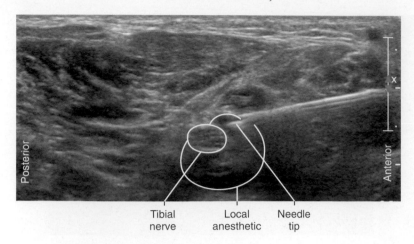

Posterior

Anterior

Tibial
nerve

Local
anesthetic

Needle
tip

Figure 49-3. Tibial nerve block in the distal leg showing the in-plane approach from anterior to posterior. Local anesthetic surrounds the tibial nerve and separates it from the posterior tibial artery.

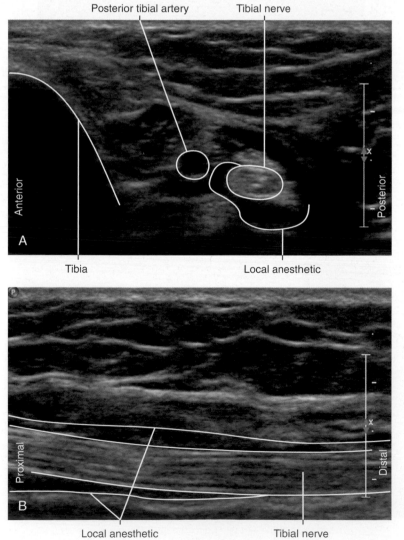

Posterior tibial artery   Tibial nerve

Anterior

Posterior

A

Tibia

Local anesthetic

Proximal

Distal

B

Local anesthetic   Tibial nerve

Figure 49-4. After injection, local anesthetic is distributed around the tibial nerve (**A**) and tracks along the nerve (**B**).

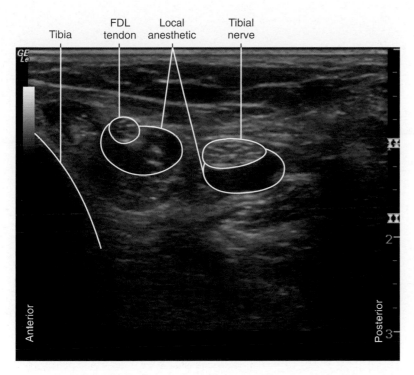

Figure 49-5. The flexor digitorum longus (FDL) tendon and tibial nerve can have similar ultrasound appearances. The flexor digitorum longus tendon is smaller than the tibial nerve and lies closer to the tibia. This sonogram was obtained after ankle block performed using surface landmarks (not ultrasound guidance). Local anesthetic is seen to surround both the tibial nerve and the flexor digitorum longus tendon.

Trunk Blocks

CHAPTER 50

INTERCOSTAL NERVE BLOCK

There are 12 pairs of intercostal nerves that lie within or near the inferior groove of each corresponding rib. These nerves supply the skin and chest wall skeletal muscles. An intercostal artery and vein accompany each nerve and lie superior to it. Intercostal nerves are difficult to image with ultrasound because they are small and often covered by the caudal edge of the corresponding rib.[1,2] Proximal intercostal nerves are found in the classic subcostal position in 17%, in the midzone in 73%, and in the inferior supracostal position in 10% of anatomic specimens.[3] The intercostal nerves migrate away from the ribs near the midaxillary line. Doppler ultrasound has been used to locate intercostal arteries for intercostal block.[4] Ultrasound-guided intercostal nerve block has been used for acute and chronic pain management.[5]

The subcostal nerve is the anterior ramus of the spinal nerve T12. This nerve supplies the lower abdominal wall and is not closely associated with the 12th rib. The subcostal nerve is about 3 mm in diameter and passes over the iliac crest.[6]

Suggested Technique

Intercostal nerve imaging can be performed in the sitting, lateral, or prone position. The arms are forward to retract the scapulae laterally. It is particularly difficult to image the intercostal nerves above the fifth rib because of the overlying scapula and paraspinous muscles. When intercostal blocks are performed in sitting position, the right-handed operator stands and turns to the patient's right to view the imaging display regardless of the side of the block.

The transducer is placed slightly medial to the posterior angulation of the ribs. In this location, the nerves are shallow and relatively centrally located before branching. This also gives the block needle room to clear the inferior rib for in-plane approach. Because of the caudal angulation of the ribs, the transducer has a slight oblique orientation, with the transducer and block needle directed slightly away from the midline. Hand-on-needle approach provides optimal needle control for intercostal blocks.

Sonograms can sometimes demonstrate three layers of the intercostal muscles (external, internal, and innermost) covering the pleural line.[7] The neurovascular bundle lies between the internal and innermost intercostal muscles. Intercostal interspaces have a flying-bat appearance on ultrasound scans because of acoustic shadowing of the ribs.[8]

For intercostal block, the needle tip is placed near the caudal edge of the rib so that the needle tip can be identified between the acoustic shadows from the bone. If the needle tip is place in the correct layer, the local anesthetic will easily track under the rib. To do this, advance the needle tip near the edge of the muscle and inject as the needle is withdrawn (similar to rectus sheath blocks). Needle tip visibility is essential for this procedure.

With intercostal nerve blocks, rapid and high peak plasma levels of local anesthetic are expected. Therefore, careful attention to drug dosing is essential. One of the potential benefits of ultrasound guidance is reduction of the risk for pneumothorax. The chance of developing a pneumothorax depends on the amount of aerated lung tissue traversed by the needle. The lung is particularly fragile in patients with chronic obstructive lung disease and emphysema. Postinterventional lung sliding and comet-tail artifact from the pleura rule out pneumothorax. This examination is best performed in the nondependent portion of the lung (the anterior chest in supine position).

Another potential benefit of ultrasound guidance for intercostal block is the avoidance of arterial puncture. This complication can result in hemothorax. This is particularly noteworthy because the tracking between the lower border of the ribs and the neurovascular bundle is not always precise. There is variability of the relationship between the caudal edge of the ribs and the neurovascular bundle, especially at the lower rib levels and further from the paravertebral region.[3]

Clinical Pearls

- The easiest patient position to perform the block is prone, but lateral or sitting is also possible.
- Intercostal blocks are best performed near the posterior angulation of the ribs. In this location, the nerves are shallow and relatively centrally located before branching.
- With intercostal nerve blocks, rapid and high peak plasma levels of local anesthetic are expected. Therefore, careful attention to drug dosing is essential.
- Because of the potential risk for pneumothorax, the intercostal nerve block technique is best learned on patients who need chest tube placement.
- Even with needle puncture of the pleura, the chance of pneumothorax is about 50%. This chance depends on the amount of aerated lung tissue traversed by the needle. The lung is particularly fragile in patients with chronic obstructive lung disease and emphysema.
- The tracking between the lower border of the ribs and the neurovascular bundle is not always perfect. Discrepancies are sometimes seen along the course of the rib.
- One of the benefits of ultrasound guidance for intercostal block is the avoidance of arterial puncture. This complication can result in hemothorax.
- Intercostal nerve blocks are useful for breast surgery and are best placed at T3, T4, and T5 for this procedure.

References

1. Peer S, Bodner G, eds. *High-Resolution Sonography of the Peripheral Nervous System.* Berlin: Springer Verlag; 2003.
2. Eichenberger U, Greher M, Curatolo M. Ultrasound in interventional pain management. *Tech Reg Anesth Pain Manag.* 2004;8:171-178.
3. Hardy PA. Anatomical variation in the position of the proximal intercostal nerve. *Br J Anaesth.* 1988;61:338-339.
4. Vaghadia H, Jenkins LC. Use of a Doppler ultrasound stethoscope for intercostal nerve block. *Can J Anaesth.* 1988;35:86-89.
5. Byas-Smith MG, Gulati A. Ultrasound-guided intercostal nerve cryoablation. *Anesth Analg.* 2006;103:1033-1035.
6. Chou D, Storm PB, Campbell JN. Vulnerability of the subcostal nerve to injury during bone graft harvesting from the iliac crest. *J Neurosurg Spine.* 2004;1:87-89.
7. Sakai F, Sone S, Kiyono K, et al. High-resolution ultrasound of the chest wall. *Rofo.* 1990;153:390-394.
8. Lichtenstein DA, Mezière G, Lascols N, et al. Ultrasound diagnosis of occult pneumothorax. *Crit Care Med.* 2005;33:1231-1238.

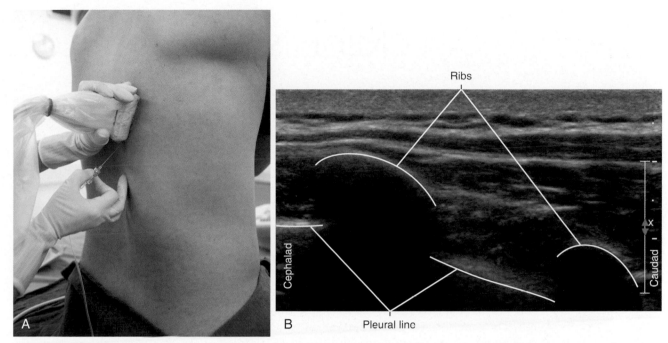

Figure 50-1. External photograph showing the approach to intercostal nerve block in sitting position (**A**). The corresponding sonogram of the intercostal interspace before needle placement is shown (**B**)

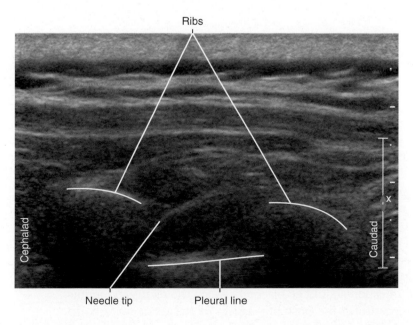

Figure 50-2. In-plane approach to intercostal nerve block. The needle tip advances between the ribs to place local anesthetic underneath the caudal edge of the superior rib.

CHAPTER 51

RECTUS SHEATH BLOCK

The rectus abdominis is a vertical muscle of the anterior abdominal wall. The muscle is divided into compartments by the midline linea alba, paramedian linea semilunaris, and transverse fibrous bands.[1] Muscles of the lateral abdominal wall (the external oblique, internal oblique, and transversus abdominis) become aponeurotic as they approach the midline. The rectus sheath consists of the rectus abdominis muscles surrounded by these aponeuroses.

Above the arcuate line, the transversalis fascia and the aponeuroses separate the rectus abdominis muscle from the abdominal cavity. Caudal to the arcuate line, the rectus abdominis muscle is in direct contact with the transversalis fascia. In this location, all three of the lateral abdominal wall muscles (external oblique, internal oblique, and transversus) have their aponeuroses pass anterior to the rectus abdominis muscle.[2]

Anterior cutaneous branches of the intercostal nerves enter the rectus sheath from the posterior and lateral side.[3] Epigastric arteries and veins are sometimes identified within the rectus sheath. The anterior intercostal nerves can run alongside these vessels before rising to the surface through the rectus abdominis muscle. The nerves of the rectus sheath are too small to be directly imaged with ultrasound.

Rectus sheath block is useful as part of a combined anesthetic technique for outpatients.[4,5] The usual indication for this block is to provide pain relief after repair of umbilical or incisional hernias. It provides an excellent alternative to straight general anesthesia or epidural blocks for surgical procedures around the midline of the abdominal wall.

Suggested Technique

The rectus sheath block is usually performed after induction of general anesthesia for patient comfort and to reduce movement. The choice of ultrasound transducer is not critical to the success of the procedure. With the patient in supine position, an in-plane approach from the lateral side of the patient is used, with the rectus abdominis muscle imaged in short-axis view (transverse). Hand-on-needle will provide excellent needle control. Tidal movement of the abdominal cavity with respiration or contraction of the abdominal wall muscles can make the procedure challenging.

The goal is to have the injected local anesthetic layer underneath the rectus abdominis muscle where the anterior intercostal nerves enter the rectus sheath. The transversalis fascia and aponeurosis of the transversus muscle form a double-layer appearance on ultrasound scans. Therefore, the needle tip and injection should be placed between the rectus abdominis muscle and the double layer that constitutes the posterior aspect of the rectus sheath. To accomplish this view, the cephalocaudad placement of the transducer should be adjusted away from tendons to allow visualization of the double layer of the transversalis fascia.

Because the nerves enter the sheath from the lateral side, the lateral aspect of the rectus abdominis muscle is targeted. The lateral edge of the rectus sheath is a potentially safer approach because it is over the abdominal wall muscles rather than the abdominal cavity. Injection of a small volume of local anesthetic on pullback of the needle through the rectus abdominis muscle will give more complete distributions.

Because of the compartmental nature of the rectus abdominis muscle, two or four injections are usually performed for periumbilical surgery (right and left sides, and sometimes above and below the umbilicus). About 5 to 10 mL of local anesthetic is injected per side per compartment in adult patients. Because the tendinous inscriptions of the muscles are not complete posteriorly,[6] some communication between compartments is possible. If local anesthetic is observed to distribute between compartments, no further injection is necessary.

The superior and inferior epigastric arteries anastomose through a vascular network. It is unlikely that large epigastric arteries will be found in the umbilical region because the contributing vessels course from above or below. Because of the lack of underlying bone, visible arterial pulsations are difficult to elicit with probe compression during rectus sheath blocks. Color Doppler can be useful during these procedures to confirm vascular identity.

Clinical Pearls

- The extent to which the abdominal wall muscles underlie the lateral corner of the rectus abdominis muscle is variable. In some cases, there is no underlying muscle to separate the rectus from the abdominal cavity.
- The needle tip should be scratched against the double layer but not actually puncture it so as to place the tip between the rectus muscle and the double layer.
- A few milliliters of local anesthetic can be injected as the needle is removed to cover the path of nerves through the rectus muscle.
- The best way to perform rectus sheath blocks is to inject forward on one side and back for the contralateral side. In this fashion, the screen and operator remain in one position for bilateral injections.
- The inferior epigastric artery has a variable position within the rectus sheath.[7]
- The fibers of the rectus abdominis course in a parallel direction, with the muscle divided by transverse tendinous intersections.[8]
- Because the nerves of the rectus sheath are small to image directly, assumptions regarding nerve position with respect to other structures must be made.
- The rectus abdominis muscle is slightly narrower near its ends at the xiphoid process and pubic bone. The rectus sheath narrows at its cephalad and caudad ends as the linea semilunaris tapers toward the midline.

References

1. Ali QM. Sonographic anatomy of the rectus sheath: an indication for new terminology and implications for rectus flaps. *Surg Radiol Anat*. 1993;15:349-353.
2. Monkhouse WS, Khalique A. Variations in the composition of the human rectus sheath: a study of the anterior abdominal wall. *J Anat*. 1986;145:61-66.
3. Rozen WM, Tran TM, Ashton MW, et al. Refining the course of the thoracolumbar nerves: a new understanding of the innervation of the anterior abdominal wall. *Clin Anat*. 2008;21:325-333.
4. Willschke H, Bösenberg A, Marhofer P, et al. Ultrasonography-guided rectus sheath block in paediatric anaesthesia: a new approach to an old technique. *Br J Anaesth*. 2006;97:244-249.
5. Sandeman DJ, Dilley AV. Ultrasound-guided rectus sheath block and catheter placement. *Aust N Z J Surg*. 2008;78:621-623.
6. Connell D, Ali K, Javid M, et al. Sonography and MRI of rectus abdominis muscle strain in elite tennis players. *AJR Am J Roentgenol*. 2006;187:1457-1461.
7. Petrossian E, Menegus MA, Issenberg HJ, et al. Ultrasound evaluation of the inferior epigastric artery. *Ann Thorac Surg*. 1994;57:895-898.
8. Erickson SJ. High-resolution imaging of the musculoskeletal system. *Radiology*. 1997;205:593-618.

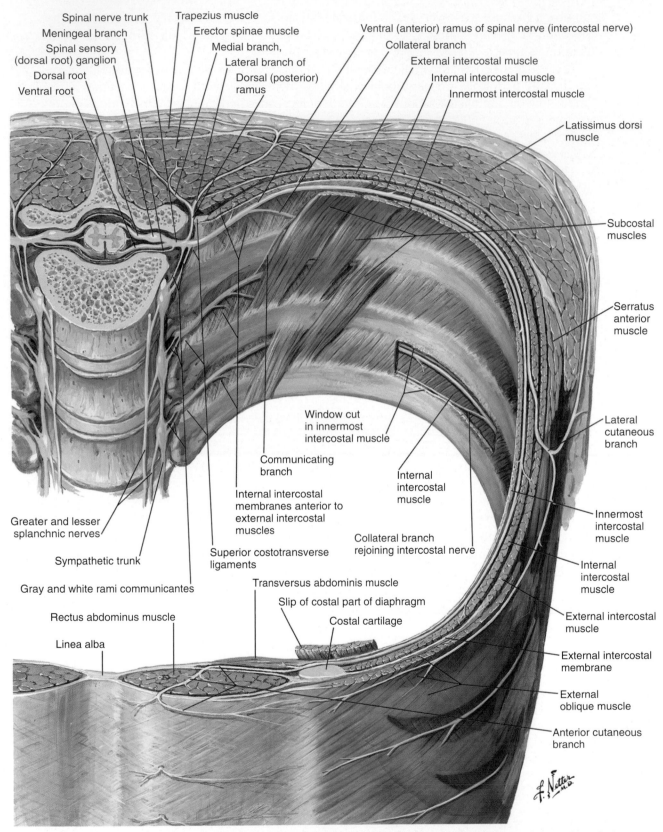

Figure 51-1. Thoracoabdominal nerves. Note the path of the anterior cutaneous branch of the intercostal nerve through the rectus abdominis muscle. (From netterimages.com, with permission.)

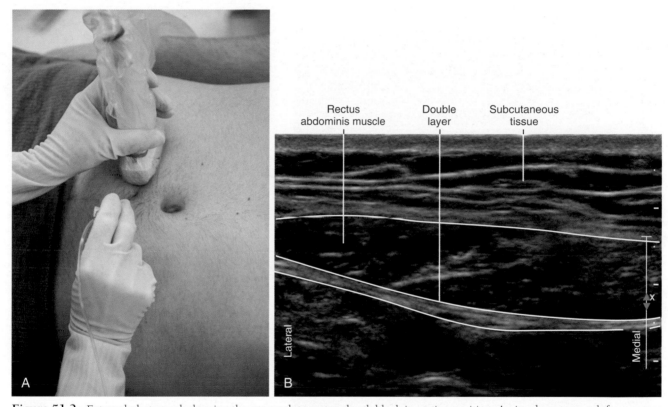

Figure 51-2. External photograph showing the approach to rectus sheath block in supine position. An in-plane approach from across the midline is shown (**A**). The corresponding sonogram in shown (**B**). The best way to perform rectus sheath blocks on both sides of the midline is to inject forward on one side compartment and back for the opposite side with the screen and operator in one position.

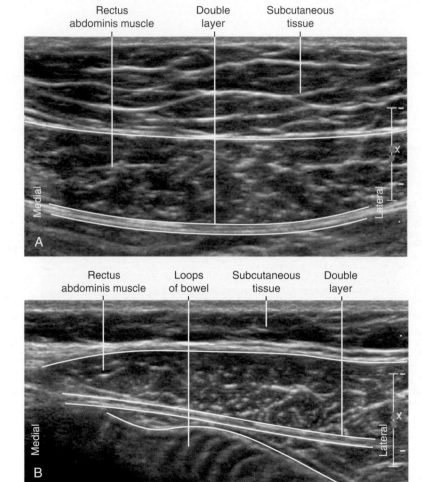

Figure 51-3. The double-layer sign indicating presence of the aponeurosis of the transversus abdominis and transversalis fascia in transverse view (**A**). Closer to the midline, loops of bowel are visualized (**B**).

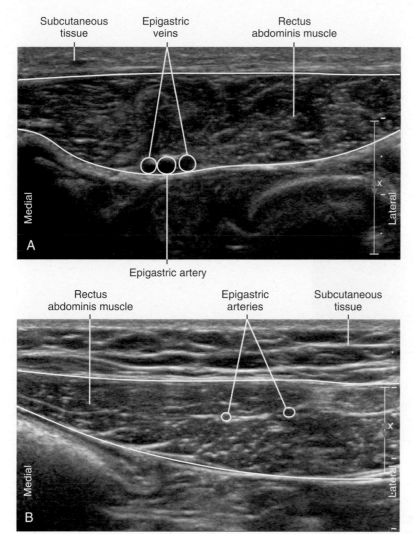

Figure 51-4. The epigastric arteries have variable position within the rectus sheath. In these examples from different patients, the arteries are seen either below (**A**) or within (**B**) the rectus sheath in transverse view.

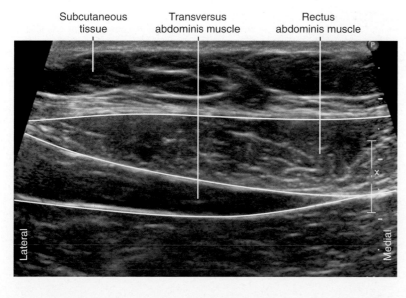

Figure 51-5. The transversus muscle on the lateral edge of the rectus abdominis in transverse view. The extent to which the abdominal wall muscles underlie the lateral corner of the rectus abdominis muscle is variable. In some cases, there is no underlying muscle to separate the rectus from the abdominal cavity.

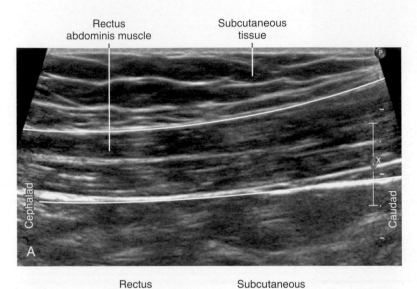

Rectus abdominis muscle   Subcutaneous tissue

Cephalad   Caudad

A

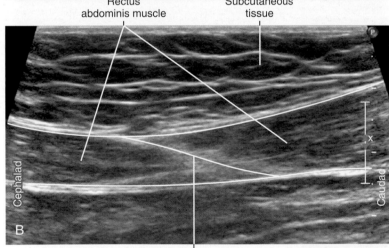

Rectus abdominis muscle   Subcutaneous tissue

Cephalad   Caudad

B

Tendinous intersection

Figure 51-6. Longitudinal views of the rectus abdominis muscle within a single muscular compartment (**A**) and in separate rectus compartments (**B**). The fibers of the rectus abdominis course in a parallel direction, with the muscle divided by transverse tendinous intersections that are typically incomplete posteriorly.

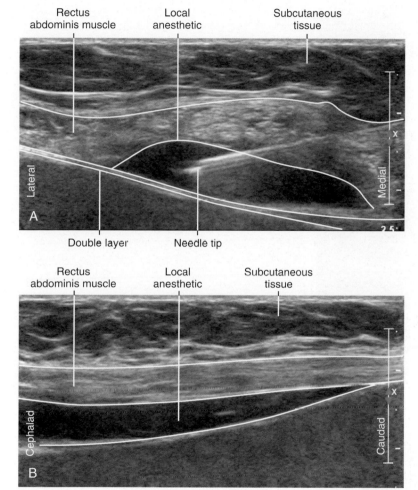

Rectus abdominis muscle   Local anesthetic   Subcutaneous tissue

Lateral

Medial

A

Double layer   Needle tip

Rectus abdominis muscle   Local anesthetic   Subcutaneous tissue

Cephalad

Caudad

B

Figure 51-7. Image sequence showing rectus sheath block. An in-plane approach is demonstrated where the needle tip is placed between the rectus muscle and the double layer (**A**). Before injection, the needle tip is gently scratched against the double layer so as to place the tip between the rectus muscle and the double layer. Local anesthetic is seen to layer underneath the muscle, giving a swimming pool appearance of successful rectus sheath injection in transverse view. A few milliliters of local anesthetic can be injected as the needle is removed to cover the path of nerves through the rectus muscle. The corresponding longitudinal view is shown (**B**).

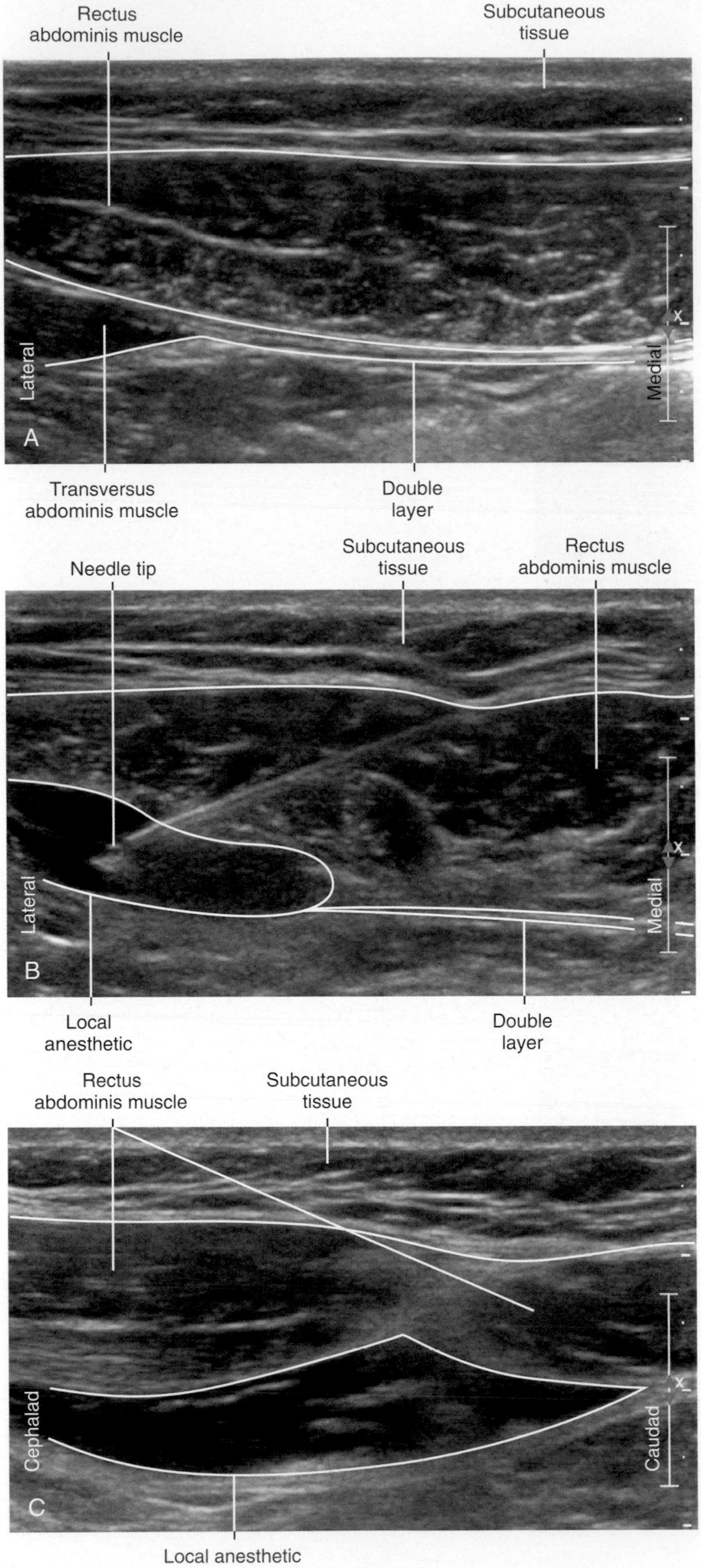

Figure 51-8. Image sequence showing rectus sheath block. Before needle tip placement, the double layer is identified (**A**). An in-plane approach is demonstrated where the needle tip and local anesthetic are placed between the rectus muscle and the double layer (**B**). After rectus sheath injection, longitudinal views can be used to assess the distribution (**C**). The handlebar moustache appearance verifies that local anesthetic has distributed to the adjacent compartment of the rectus abdominis muscle.

CHAPTER 52

ILIOINGUINAL NERVE BLOCK

The anterior and lateral abdominal wall is primarily supplied by the subcostal, iliohypogastric, ilioinguinal, and genitofemoral nerves. The latter three nerves arise from the lumbar plexus. Ilioinguinal nerve blocks are often performed to provide postoperative pain relief from inguinal hernia repair.

The iliohypogastric and ilioinguinal nerves cross the anterior surface of the quadratus lumborum before piercing the transversus abdominis muscle. The quadratus lumborum (rather than the abdominal cavity) lies under the abdominal wall muscles between the costal margin and the pelvic brim when imaging posterior and lateral. Medially, the transversalis fascia separates the transversus muscle from the peritoneal cavity.

The ilioinguinal nerve emerges between the muscles of the abdominal wall. The longest running course of the nerve is between the internal oblique and transversus muscles. The iliohypogastric nerve has a parallel course to the ilioinguinal nerve, running cephalad (superior) and medial. Of the three abdominal wall muscles (external oblique, internal oblique, and transversus), the internal oblique is the thickest.[1]

The deep (medial) circumflex artery is a branch of the external iliac artery. The deep circumflex artery pierces the transversus as it ascends the abdominal wall. Branches of the deep circumflex iliac artery often accompany the ilioinguinal nerves.

Suggested Technique

Nerve and muscle visibility are best cephalad to the pelvic brim.[2] In the classic location for ilioinguinal block (2 cm medial and 2 cm superior to the anterior-superior iliac spine), the external oblique muscle is often aponeurotic, and therefore it is difficult to visualize this layer over the nerves. The first step is to obtain a view of the three abdominal wall muscles (external oblique, internal oblique, and transversus) to identify the ilioinguinal nerves between the internal oblique and transversus. Alternatively, the deep circumflex artery can be followed up from the external iliac artery until it meets the ilioinguinal nerves.

One approach is to perform the block across midline (across the table). The block needle approaches in-plane from medial to lateral to steer away from the abdominal cavity. The needle tip should be positioned between the internal oblique and transversus muscles. Local anesthetic should layer between the two muscles to block multiple nerves.[3] Because the in-plane approach has a shallow angle, the block needle has a tendency to skim over the fascia rather than pierce it.

Clinical Pearls

- Ilioinguinal blocks are useful for pain relief after lower abdominal incisions (e.g., cesarean delivery, abdominal hysterectomy) and inguinal hernia repair.
- The course of the ilioinguinal nerve and deep circumflex iliac artery parallels the inside aspect of the pelvic brim.[4]
- The needle should be aimed at the corner of the neurovascular bundle, where the ilioinguinal nerves lie adjacent to the deep circumflex iliac artery. Color or power Doppler helps identify this artery. In contrast to the artery, the nerves will not have color encoding. At the levels of compression for imaging, the adjacent veins should be collapsed. The injection can be performed where the artery lies between the internal oblique and transversus muscle layers or as proximal as possible.[5]
- The transversus muscle is thin, and therefore intraperitoneal placement of the needle tip has occurred during ilioinguinal blocks.[6]
- The diameters of the ilioinguinal and iliohypogastric nerves are about 3 by 1.5 mm each. The two nerves usually lie about 10 mm apart from each other. The ilioinguinal nerve lies about 6 mm from the iliac bone. One common anatomic variation in this region is fusion of the ilioinguinal and iliohypogastric nerves into a common trunk, occurring in about 12% of normal subjects.[2]
- The best imaging of these nerves is about 5 cm cranial and slightly posterior to the anterior-superior iliac spine. In this location, the two nerves consistently lie between the internal oblique and transversus muscles.[2]
- The transducer should be slightly rotated to image perpendicular to the course of the nerves and close enough to the bone that the iliac crest should be within the field of view. If the needle tip is sufficiently lateral, the iliacus or quadratus lumborum muscle, rather than peritoneum, will lie under the transversus.
- Because the cutaneous innervation of the ilioinguinal nerves is variable, there are no accurate clinical tests of assessment.

References

1. Rankin G, Stokes M, Newham DJ. Abdominal muscle size and symmetry in normal subjects. *Muscle Nerve*. 2006;34:320-326.
2. Eichenberger U, Greher M, Kirchmair L, et al. Ultrasound-guided blocks of the ilioinguinal and iliohypogastric nerve: accuracy of a selective new technique confirmed by anatomical dissection. *Br J Anaesth*. 2006;97:238-243.
3. Hebbard P, Fujiwara Y, Shibata Y, Royse C. Ultrasound-guided transversus abdominis plane (TAP) block. *Anaesth Intensive Care*. 2007;35:616-617.
4. Schlenz I, Burggasser G, Kuzbari R, et al. External oblique abdominal muscle: a new look on its blood supply and innervation. *Anat Rec*. 1999;255:388-395.
5. Tran TM, Ivanusic JJ, Hebbard P, Barrington MJ. Determination of spread of injectate after ultrasound-guided transversus abdominis plane block: a cadaveric study. *Br J Anaesth*. 2009;102:123-127.
6. Jankovic Z, Ahmad N, Ravishankar N, Archer F. Transversus abdominis plane block: how safe is it? *Anesth Analg*. 2008; 107:1758-1759.

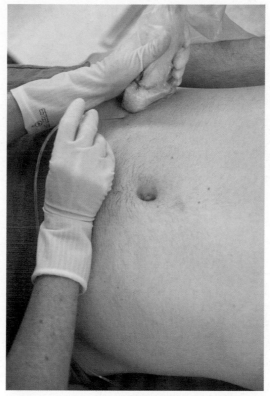

Figure 52-1. External photograph showing the in-plane approach to ilioinguinal nerve block above the iliac crest.

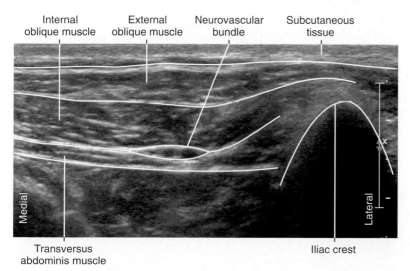

Internal oblique muscle   External oblique muscle   Neurovascular bundle   Subcutaneous tissue

Medial

Lateral

Transversus abdominis muscle   Iliac crest

Figure 52-2. Sonogram showing the neurovascular bundle between the internal oblique and transversus muscles adjacent to the iliac bone.

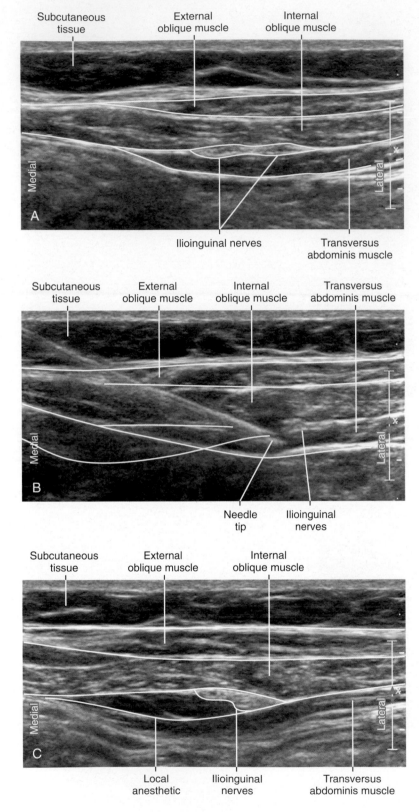

A

Subcutaneous tissue
External oblique muscle
Internal oblique muscle
Ilioinguinal nerves
Transversus abdominis muscle
Medial
Lateral

B

Subcutaneous tissue
External oblique muscle
Internal oblique muscle
Transversus abdominis muscle
Needle tip
Ilioinguinal nerves
Medial
Lateral

C

Subcutaneous tissue
External oblique muscle
Internal oblique muscle
Local anesthetic
Ilioinguinal nerves
Transversus abdominis muscle
Medial
Lateral

Figure 52-3. Image sequence showing ilioinguinal nerve block. Sonogram demonstrating the ilioinguinal nerves before needle placement (**A**). An in-plane approach is demonstrated where the needle tip is placed in the fascial layer between the internal oblique and transversus muscles adjacent to the nerves (**B**). After injection, local anesthetic layers next to the ilioinguinal nerves (**C**).

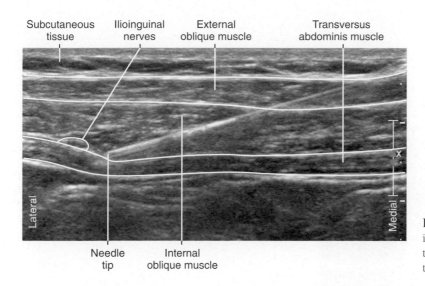

Subcutaneous tissue   Ilioinguinal nerves   External oblique muscle   Transversus abdominis muscle

Lateral

Medial

Needle tip   Internal oblique muscle

Figure 52-4. Soft tissue properties are important during ilioinguinal block. During in-plane approach, the needle tip will compress the soft tissue substantially before puncturing the muscle layer.

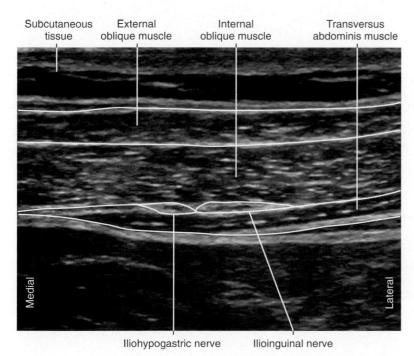

Subcutaneous tissue   External oblique muscle   Internal oblique muscle   Transversus abdominis muscle

Medial

Lateral

Iliohypogastric nerve   Ilioinguinal nerve

Figure 52-5. In some patients, both the ilioinguinal and iliohypogastric nerves can be identified between the internal oblique and transversus muscles. The nerves usually lie 1 cm apart, but substantial variability exists.

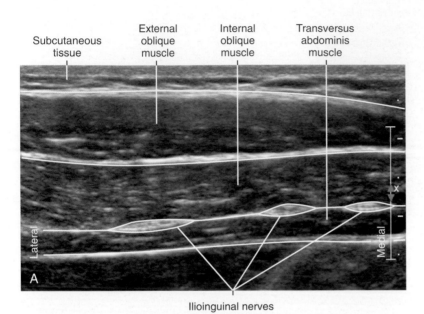

Subcutaneous tissue   External oblique muscle   Internal oblique muscle   Transversus abdominis muscle

Lateral

Medial

A

Ilioinguinal nerves

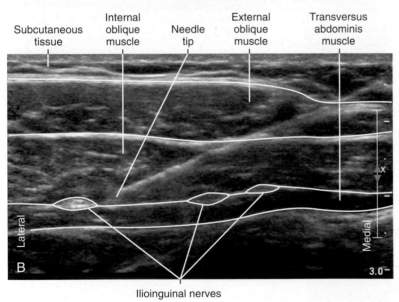

Subcutaneous tissue   Internal oblique muscle   Needle tip   External oblique muscle   Transversus abdominis muscle

Lateral

Medial

B

3.0

Ilioinguinal nerves

Figure 52-6. In rare patients, three nerves (here collectively referred to as ilioinguinal nerves) can be identified between the internal oblique and transversus muscles (**A**). Corresponding sonogram during regional block (**B**). The needle tip is placed in the fascial layer between the identified nerves.

CHAPTER 53

NEURAXIAL BLOCK

In many patients, epidural and spinal blocks are routine procedures guided by loss of resistance and confirmation of free flow of cerebrospinal fluid, respectively. However, in patients with obesity or advanced age, these neuraxial blocks can be more challenging and may benefit from imaging guidance. Ultrasound imaging has been reported useful for guiding neuraxial anesthetics in patients with prior surgical instrumentation or scoliosis.[1,2] Ultrasound can estimate the location and level of spinous interspaces. The first description of ultrasound imaging of the epidural space was in 1980.[3] However, there remain current limitations to the use of ultrasound technology to guide neuraxial blocks.

Neuraxial imaging with ultrasound is difficult because of the depth of the structures of interest and the surrounding bone. The narrow acoustic window makes on-line approaches inherently challenging. Simultaneous ultrasound imaging and needle placement for neuraxial procedures are difficult in adult patients. On-line approaches to neuraxial procedures are more commonly used in pediatric patients.[4,5]

Selection of the correct interspace is important to the success of subarachnoid block. The interspace selected for injection of spinal anesthetic drugs affects the resultant distribution. The failure rate at lower lumbar interspaces can be as high as 7%.[6,7] One of the potential benefits of ultrasound is to help establish the correct interspace for neuraxial block.

The accuracy of ultrasonography in correctly identifying lumbar interspace levels is in the 71% to 76% range for patients undergoing magnetic resonance imaging to evaluate the lumbar spine.[8,9] The ability to estimate the interspace level is especially complex in patients with transitional vertebrae. These anomalies include lumbarization of the sacral spine (an unfused first sacral vertebra) and sacralization of the lumbar spine (fusion of L5 with the sacrum).[10] The number of ribs also can vary, making estimation of level relative to the thoracic vertebrae challenging.[11] Although ultrasound has limited ability to assess the interspace level, assessment by palpation is more inaccurate.[12]

Suggested Technique

Off-line imaging can be performed in the same position as used for procedures without imaging guidance. Prone or lateral position is optimal for on-line technique. With lateral position, the block needle approaches from the nondependent side toward the midline.

Ultrasound is an accurate imaging modality for depiction of the dura mater.[13] The dura appears highly echogenic on ultrasound scans, defined by a typical double-layer hyperechoic signal.[14] The subarachnoid space is distensible. Dural tenting during combined spinal-epidural procedures has been estimated to be 2.4 mm.[15] The width of the subarachnoid space is about 15 mm. Hydrostatic forces cause a 1- to 2-mm increase in diameter with postural changes from supine to sitting.[16] Because the subarachnoid space contains few endogenous scatterers of ultrasound, it appears echo free on ultrasound scans.

Paramedian longitudinal imaging planes are generally preferred for visualization of neur-axial structures.[17] With this view, the width of the acoustic window (the intervertebral space) is largest relative to the shadowing of the corresponding vertebral bone. This view is typically used to select an interspace for regional block by including the sacrum in the view as a refer-ence point. Several authors have described the epidural space to have a sawtooth configura-tion in sagittal or parasagittal view.[18]

Some advocate additional use of the transverse view after marking the interspace level.[19,20] Transverse view has been described as having a flying-bat appearance. The transverse view of a lumbar interspace has been described as resembling a flying bat (to be distinguished from the flying-bat sign of the intercostal interspaces).[21] In the midline of the interspace, a hyperechoic band corresponding to the ligamentum flavum and the dorsal dura is visualized (the head of the bat). A second, deeper hyperechoic band, parallel to the first band, corre-sponds to the anterior dura, the posterior longitudinal ligament, and the vertebral body. In addition, paramedian hyperechoic structures, corresponding to the articular and transverse processes, are also visualized through the acoustic window (the ears or wings of the bat).

Limitations of off-line technique (skin markings before needle placement) are severalfold. First, it can be difficult to estimate the angle of approach for the needle from the transducer orientation. The needle trajectory for subarachnoid block (or epidural placement) is expected to be in the range of 10 to 30 degrees.[22] Second, skin mobility makes it possible for the skin markings to be displaced from the correct location. Third, changes in patient positioning can occur between the time of skin markings and the actual procedure. Finally, the soft tissue dynamics of needle placement can only be appreciated with on-line techniques. The estima-tion of depth and angle for needle placement from off-line sonograms is a complex matter involving many factors.

Concerns have been raised regarding potential toxicity of acoustic coupling gel if inadver-tently introduced into the subarachnoid space. However, live ultrasound has been used for lumbar puncture and epidural placement in thousands of pediatric cases without apparent problems of gel toxicity.[4,5]

Clinical Pearls

- The saw sign of paramedian longitudinal views inclines toward the skin surface in the caudal direction.
- Although transverse plane imaging has been shown to be effective at lumbar inter-spaces, it is not helpful at mid-thoracic levels because of the narrower acoustic windows across the midline. Whether transverse plane imaging is effective at low thoracic levels remains to be established.
- Mark the location, depth, and interspace on the back. Because the skin is less mobile on the back, skin markings have greater utility.
- The parallel hyperechoic bands consist of the ligamentum flavum and posterior dura (shallow) and the anterior dura, posterior longitudinal ligament, and vertebral body (deep).
- The needle follows the same angle for optimal visualization of the neuraxis.
- It can be difficult to obtain symmetrical views of the neuraxis (in particular, the articular processes) in patients with scoliosis due to rotation of the spine.
- Note that off-line distance measurements can underestimate true distances in part because of tissue compression during scanning (also due to subcutaneous local anesthetic infiltration and needle tenting and deformation of soft tissue), although measurements are typically accurate to within 1 cm. However, this trend toward underestimation was not born out in a recent study of labor epidural placement.[19]
- Loss of resistance is visualized as widening of the epidural space followed by ventral movement of the dural cover and compression of the dural sac.[5]

References

1. Yeo ST, French R. Combined spinal-epidural in the obstetric patient with Harrington rods assisted by ultrasonography. *Br J Anaesth*. 1999;83:670-672.
2. McLeod A, Roche A, Fennelly M. Case series: ultrasonography may assist epidural insertion in scoliosis patients. *Can J Anaesth*. 2005;52:717-720.
3. Cork RC, Kryc JJ, Vaughan RW. Ultrasonic localization of the lumbar epidural space. *Anesthesiology*. 1980;52:513-516.
4. Coley BD, Murakami JW, Koch BL, et al. Diagnostic and interventional ultrasound of the pediatric spine. *Pediatr Radiol*. 2001;31:775-785.
5. Rapp HJ, Folger A, Grau T. Ultrasound-guided epidural catheter insertion in children. *Anesth Analg*. 2005;101:333-339.
6. Munhall RJ, Sukhani R, Winnie AP. Incidence and etiology of failed spinal anesthetics in a university hospital: a prospective study. *Anesth Analg*. 1988;67:843-848.
7. Tarkkila PJ. Incidence and causes of failed spinal anesthetics in a university hospital: a prospective study. *Reg Anesth*. 1991;16:48-51.
8. Furness G, Reilly MP, Kuchi S. An evaluation of ultrasound imaging for identification of lumbar intervertebral level. *Anaesthesia*. 2002;57:277-280.
9. Watson MJ, Evans S, Thorp JM. Could ultrasonography be used by an anaesthetist to identify a specified lumbar interspace before spinal anaesthesia? *Br J Anaesth*. 2003;90:509-511.
10. Hahn PY, Strobel JJ, Hahn FJ. Verification of lumbosacral segments on MR images: identification of transitional vertebrae. *Radiology*. 1992;182:580-581.
11. Glass RB, Norton KI, Mitre SA, Kang E. Pediatric ribs: a spectrum of abnormalities. *Radiographics*. 2002;22:87-104.
12. Kim JT, Bahk JH, Sung J. Influence of age and sex on the position of the conus medullaris and Tuffier's line in adults. *Anesthesiology*. 2003;99:1359-1363.
13. Grau T, Leipold RW, Delorme S, et al. Ultrasound imaging of the thoracic epidural space. *Reg Anesth Pain Med*. 2002;27:200-206.
14. Rapp HJ, Grau T. Ultrasound imaging in pediatric regional anesthesia. *Can J Anaesth*. 2004;51:277-278.
15. Grau T, Leipold RW, Fatehi S, et al. Real-time ultrasonic observation of combined spinal-epidural anaesthesia. *Eur J Anaesthesiol*. 2004;21:25-31.
16. Hirasawa Y, Bashir WA, Smith FW, et al. Postural changes of the dural sac in the lumbar spines of asymptomatic individuals using positional stand-up magnetic resonance imaging. *Spine*. 2007;32:E136-E140.
17. Grau T, Leipold RW, Horter J, et al. Paramedian access to the epidural space: the optimum window for ultrasound imaging. *J Clin Anesth*. 2001;13:213-217.
18. Grau T, Leipold RW, Conradi R, Martin E. Ultrasound control for presumed difficult epidural puncture. *Acta Anaesthesiol Scand*. 2001;45:766-771.
19. Arzola C, Davies S, Rofaeel A, Carvalho JC. Ultrasound using the transverse approach to the lumbar spine provides reliable landmarks for labor epidurals. *Anesth Analg*. 2007;104:1188-1192.
20. Carvalho JC. Ultrasound-facilitated epidurals and spinals in obstetrics. *Anesthesiol Clin*. 2008;26:145-158.
21. Lichtenstein DA, Mezière G, Lascols N, et al. Ultrasound diagnosis of occult pneumothorax. *Crit Care Med*. 2005;33:1231-1238.
22. Grau T, Leipold RW, Horter J, et al. The lumbar epidural space in pregnancy: visualization by ultrasonography. *Br J Anaesth*. 2001;86:798-804.

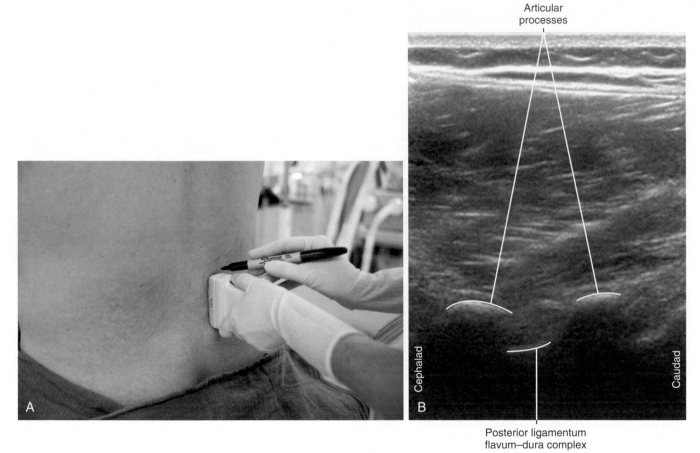

Figure 53-1. External photograph showing transducer position for paramedian view of the neuraxis and off-line technique (**A**). Corresponding sonogram demonstrates the saw sign (**B**). The saw sign represents the articular processes of the lumbar vertebrae (the teeth of the saw) and the interspaces (the spaces between the teeth). To obtain this view, the transducer is placed 2 to 3 cm off midline and tilted to the center of the spinal canal.

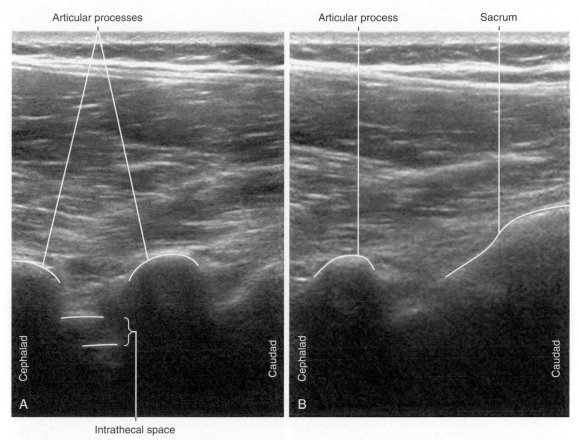

Articular processes

Articular process   Sacrum

Cephalad   Caudad

Cephalad   Caudad

A   B

Intrathecal space

Figure 53-2. Paramedian view at the lower lumbar interspaces. The acoustic window shows the spinal canal (**A**). The hyperechoic sacrum can be identified and, by inference, the L5-S1 interspace (**B**).

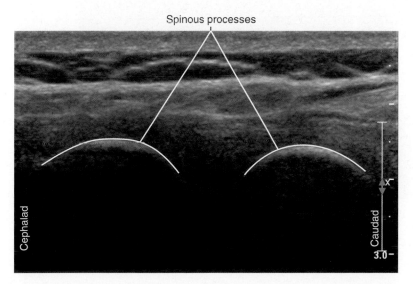

Spinous processes

Cephalad

Caudad

3.0 —

Figure 53-3. Midline longitudinal view demonstrating the spinous processes and interspace.

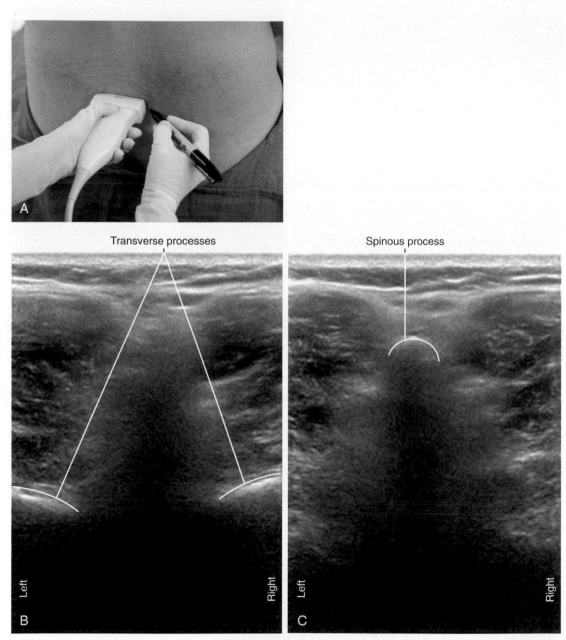

Figure 53-4. External photograph showing transducer position for transverse view of the neuraxis and off-line technique (**A**). Corresponding sonogram (**B**). If the probe is away from the interspace, the spinous process is viewed and produces an acoustic shadow (**C**).

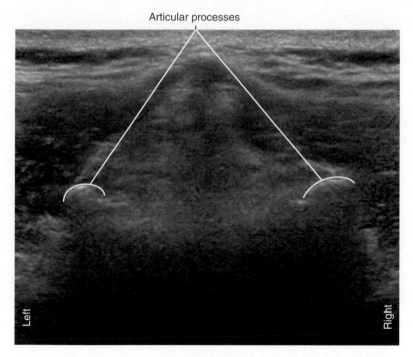

Articular processes

Left

Right

Figure 53-5. Transverse sonogram demonstrating the acoustic shadows of the articular processes.

54

CAUDAL EPIDURAL BLOCK

The spinal epidural space extends from the foramen magnum to the sacral hiatus. The caudal epidural space can be accessed through the sacrococcygeal ligament that covers the sacral hiatus. Caudal blocks provide anesthesia for genitourinary and anorectal surgical procedures. This procedure is normally performed by placing a needle or catheter through the sacrococcygeal ligament for injection of local anesthetic drugs. Unlike subarachnoid blocks, caudal blocks are relatively easy to perform in prone position. The caudal approach is usually the most superficial access to the epidural space.

The sacral hiatus is the caudal termination of the sacral canal. The volume of the epidural space within the sacral canal is highly variable, with estimates ranging from 10 to 26 mL in adults (Table 54-1).[1] In this study of 37 adults (23 female, 14 male), the sacrococcygeal membrane was significantly thicker in females than in males (mean values, 3.6 and 2.5 mm, respectively).[1] The sacral canal volume was significantly smaller in females than in males (mean values 13.2 and 16.5 mL, respectively).[1] Because the sacral canal volume varies, the dose required to achieve a given level of caudal epidural block will vary from individual to individual.

TABLE 54-1	Magnetic Resonance Imaging Estimates of Caudal Space Anatomy in Adults		
		MEAN VALUE	RANGE
Patient Data			
Height (cm)		168	150-183
Weight (kg)		72	49-120
Sacrococcygeal Membrane			
Absence (%)		10.8	
Thickness (mm)		3.2	1-5
Sacral Canal			
Maximum anteroposterior diameter (mm)		4.6	1-8
Angle (degrees)		57.9	40-74
Volume (mL)		14.4	9.5-26.6
Dural Sac			
Shortest distance from sacrococcygeal membrane to dural sac (mm)		60.5	34-80

Adapted from Crighton IM, Barry BP, Hobbs GJ. A study of the anatomy of the caudal space using magnetic resonance imaging. *Br J Anaesth.* 1997;78:391-395.

TABLE 54-2	Estimates of the Level of the Caudal Termination of the Dural Sac in Adults			
METHOD	MEDIAN LEVEL	RANGE	NO. PATIENTS	REFERENCE
Myelography	S2	S1 to S4	160	Evison et al[2] (1979)
Myelography	S1/S2	S1 (U2) to S4/S5	121	Larsen and Olsen[3] (1991)
MRI	S2	S2 to S2-3	20	Hirabayashi et al[4] (1995)
MRI	S2 (M3)	S1 (U3) to S4 (U3)	37	Crighton et al[5] (1997)
MRI	S2 (M3)	S1 (U3) to S4 (U3)	136	MacDonald et al[6] (1999)
MRI	S2 (M3)	S1 (U3) to S3 (L3)	690	Kim et al[7] (2003)
MRI	S2 (U3)	L5-S1 to S3 (U3)	743	Binokay et al[8] (2006)

U3, upper third; M3, middle third; L3, lower third; U2, upper half.

In adults, the dural sac of the subarachnoid space ends between the S1 and S2 sacral segments.[1] In this study, the distance between the dural sac and sacrococcygeal ligament ranged from 34 to 80 mm. The S5 and coccygeal nerves normally exit the sacral canal through the sacral hiatus. The sacral and coccygeal cornua (horns) articulate to form an archlike structure. Table 54-2 summarizes the estimates of the level of the caudal termination of the dural sac in adults gathered from several studies.

Variations in sacral anatomy are relatively common. A number of conditions can make caudal block difficult, including narrowing or complete absence of the sacral hiatus.[9,10] These conditions occur in 3% to 6% of anatomic specimens. The sacral cornua are prominent (>3 mm of bony prominence on each side) in only 21% of adult sacrums,[9] and therefore assessment by palpation is problematic.

The sacral epidural space is highly vascular. Inadvertent intravenous injection is relatively common during caudal block, occurring in about 5% to 10% of these procedures.[11]

Landmarks for caudal block are traditionally assessed by palpation. The posterior-superior iliac spines (the superolateral sacral crests of the sacrum) form an equilateral triangle with the sacral hiatus.[10] Although this approximation is accurate, the clinical assessment of landmark position can be difficult. Traditional techniques also rely on tactile sense of needle entry into the caudal space. However, the sacrococcygeal ligament is soft in children and may therefore not be easy to detect manually by needle advancement.[12]

Ultrasound can be used to guide caudal blocks in pediatric and adult patients.[13,14] Sonography can determine the location and size of the sacral hiatus for needle tip placement. In addition, ultrasound can be used to image the distribution after caudal epidural injection. However, the bone of the sacrum prevents ultrasound imaging of most of the sacral canal. One concern is that acoustic shadowing from the overlying bone can prevent detection of intravascular injection during caudal blocks, particularly in adults. Ultrasound imaging may be of particular utility in guiding caudal injections in patients with spinal dysraphism.[15]

Suggested Technique

Caudal block with ultrasound is optimally performed in prone position with sterile transducer cover and skin preparation. The wide variety of transducer selections for caudal block depend on patient size.[11] In thin adult patients, a 5- to 10-MHz small-footprint "hockey-stick" trans-

Clinical Pearls—cont'd

Verification of Caudal Epidural Needle Tip Placement

- Cardiac oscillations of a saline column waveform also can be used to confirm caudal epidural placement, similar to that described for other parts of the epidural space.[21]

Aspiration

- Aspirate to help rule out intravascular needle tip placement. Aspirate frequently because the caudal epidural space is highly vascular.
- Because of the overlying cornual bone, probe compression will not help identify epidural arteries and veins.

Injection

- Because caudal epidural injections have low resistance, the visible color distribution should fill the entire epidural space within the field of view.
- Caudal epidural injections can appear similar to intravascular injections with ultrasound imaging.
- Tenting of the sacrococcygeal ligament and caudal displacement of the canal are signs of correct caudal epidural injection.
- One dominant color indicates successful caudal epidural steroid injection.[19]

Air Versus Saline

- Slow injection of 2 mL air can be used to confirm needle placement in the caudal epidural space.[11] If the needle is correctly placed within the caudal epidural space, air will not be visualized outside the sacrococcygeal ligament. The volume of air is minimized to reduce the chance of unblocked segments due to air locks within the epidural space.[22,23]

Assessment

- The lateral aspect of the foot is reliably innervated by S1 for cutaneous assessment of the upper extent of sacral caudal block.

References

1. Crighton IM, Barry BP, Hobbs GJ. A study of the anatomy of the caudal space using magnetic resonance imaging. *Br J Anaesth.* 1997;78:391-395.
2. Evison G, Windsor P, Duck F. Myelographic features of the normal sacral sac. *Br J Radiol.* 1979;52:777-780.
3. Larsen JL, Olsen KO. Radiographic anatomy of the distal dural sac. A myelographic investigation of dimensions and termination. *Acta Radiol.* 1991;32:214-219.
4. Hirabayashi Y, Shimizu R, Saitoh K, et al. Anatomical configuration of the spinal column in the supine position. I. A study using magnetic resonance imaging. *Br J Anaesth.* 1995;75:3-5.
5. Crighton IM, Barry BP, Hobbs GJ. A study of the anatomy of the caudal space using magnetic resonance imaging. *Br J Anaesth.* 1997;78:391-395.
6. MacDonald A, Chatrath P, Spector T, Ellis H. Level of termination of the spinal cord and the dural sac: a magnetic resonance study. *Clin Anat.* 1999;12:149-152.
7. Kim JT, Bahk JH, Sung J. Influence of age and sex on the position of the conus medullaris and Tuffier's line in adults. *Anesthesiology.* 2003;99:1359-1363.
8. Binokay F, Akgul E, Bicakci K, et al. Determining the level of the dural sac tip: magnetic resonance imaging in an adult population. *Acta Radiol.* 2006;47:397-400.

9. Sekiguchi M, Yabuki S, Satoh K, Kikuchi S. An anatomic study of the sacral hiatus: a basis for successful caudal epidural block. *Clin J Pain.* 2004;20:51-54.
10. Senoglu N, Senoglu M, Oksuz H, et al. Landmarks of the sacral hiatus for caudal epidural block: an anatomical study. *Br J Anaesth.* 2005;95:692-695.
11. Klocke R, Jenkinson T, Glew D. Sonographically guided caudal epidural steroid injections. *J Ultrasound Med.* 2003;22:1229-1232.
12. Park JH, Koo BN, Kim JY, et al. Determination of the optimal angle for needle insertion during caudal block in children using ultrasound imaging. *Anaesthesia.* 2006;61:946-949.
13. Rapp HJ, Grau T. Ultrasound imaging in pediatric regional anesthesia. *Can J Anaesth.* 2004;51:277-278.
14. Chen CP, Tang SF, Hsu TC, et al. Ultrasound guidance in caudal epidural needle placement. *Anesthesiology.* 2004;101:181-184.
15. Roberts SA, Guruswamy V, Galvez I. Caudal injectate can be reliably imaged using portable ultrasound: a preliminary study. *Paediatr Anaesth.* 2005;15:948-952.
16. Schwartz D, Raghunathan K, Dunn S, Connelly NR. Ultrasonography and pediatric caudals. *Anesth Analg.* 2008;106:97-99.
17. Adewale L, Dearlove O, Wilson B, et al. The caudal canal in children: a study using magnetic resonance imaging. *Paediatr Anaesth.* 2000;10:137-141.
18. Beek FJ, Bax KM, Mali WP. Sonography of the coccyx in newborns and infants. *J Ultrasound Med.* 1994;13:629-634.
19. Yoon JS, Sim KH, Kim SJ, et al. The feasibility of color Doppler ultrasonography for caudal epidural steroid injection. *Pain.* 2005;118:210-214.
20. Broadman L, Ivani G. Caudal blocks. *Tech Reg Anesth Pain Med.* 1999;3:150-156.
21. Ghia JN, Arora SK, Castillo M, Mukherji SK. Confirmation of location of epidural catheters by epidural pressure waveform and computed tomography cathetergram. *Reg Anesth Pain Med.* 2001;26:337-341.
22. Dalens B, Bazin JE, Haberer JP. Epidural bubbles as a cause of incomplete analgesia during epidural anesthesia. *Anesth Analg.* 1987;66:679-683.
23. Boezaart AP, Levendig BJ. Epidural air-filled bubbles and unblocked segments. *Can J Anaesth.* 1989;36:603-604.

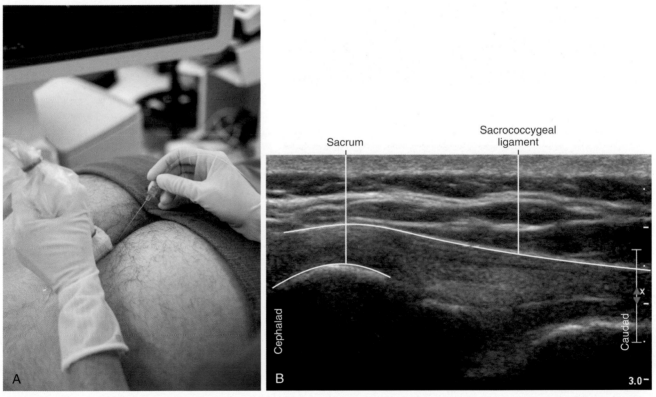

Figure 54-1. External photograph showing longitudinal in-plane approach to caudal epidural block (**A**). Corresponding sonogram obtained before needle placement (**B**). In this sonogram, the sacrococcygeal ligament can be seen overlying the sacral hiatus.

Sacral cornua

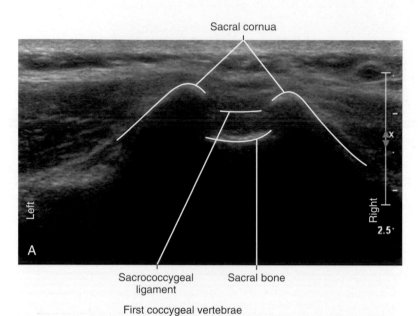

Left

Right

2.5'

A

Sacrococcygeal
ligament

Sacral bone

First coccygeal vertebrae

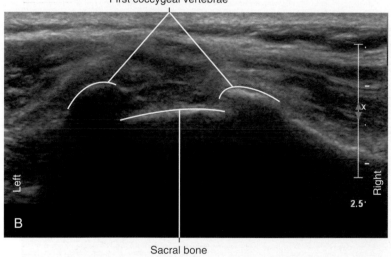

Left

Right

2.5'

B

Sacral bone

Figure 54-2. Transverse view of the sacral cornua (**A**). These bones appear as inverted U shapes in transverse view with acoustic shadowing. The hyperechoic lines between the cornua are the sacrococcygeal ligament and underlying sacral bone, with the sacral hiatus lying between these two structures. More distally, the caudal epidural space narrows as the transverse processes of the first coccygeal vertebra come into view (**B**). This indicates the transducer is caudal to the sacral hiatus.

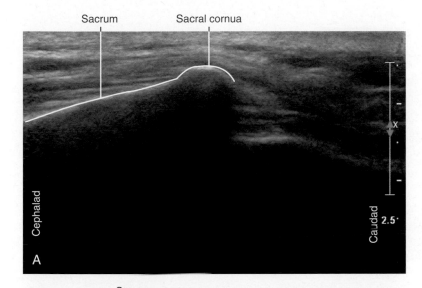

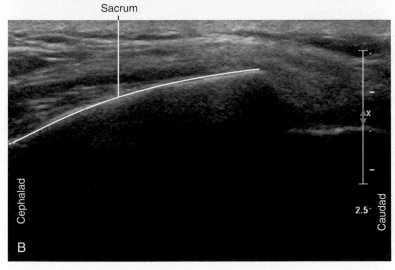

Figure 54-3. Longitudinal view of the sacrum demonstrating the presence (**A**) or absence (**B**) of the sacral cornua in the imaging plane.

Needle tip

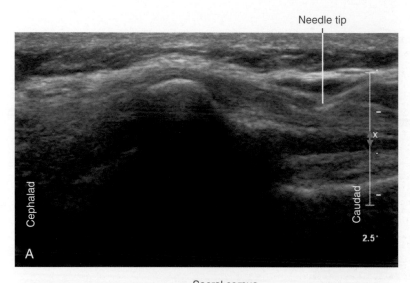

Cephalad

Caudad

2.5˚

A

Sacral cornua

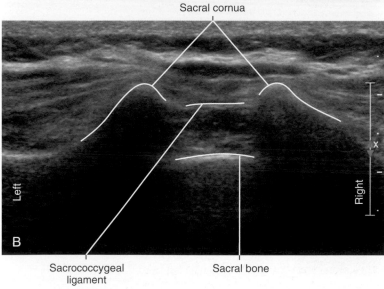

Left

Right

x

B

Sacrococcygeal
ligament

Sacral bone

Figure 54-4. Longitudinal in-plane approach to caudal epidural block (**A**). The corresponding transverse view is shown (**B**).

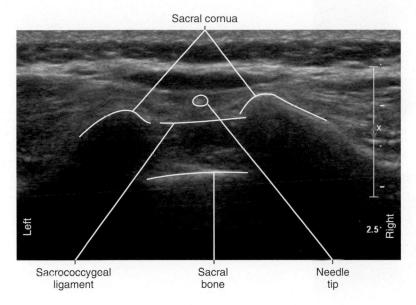

Figure 54-5. Transverse out-of-plane approach to caudal epidural block. The needle tip crosses the plane of imaging as an echogenic dot.

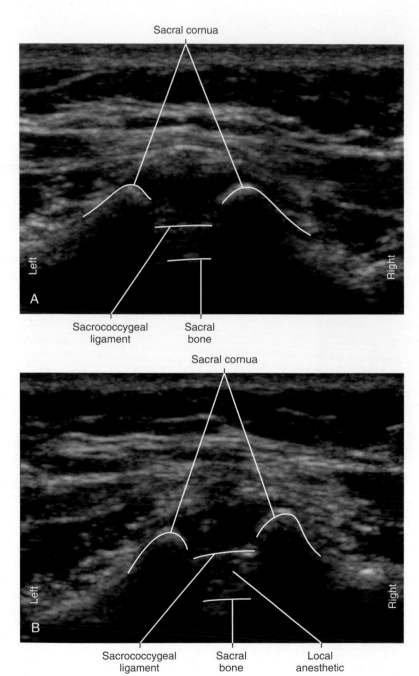

Sacral cornua

Left

Right

A

Sacrococcygeal
ligament

Sacral
bone

Sacral cornua

Left

Right

B

Sacrococcygeal
ligament

Sacral
bone

Local
anesthetic

Figure 54-6. Pediatric caudal epidural guided by ultrasound. These transverse sonograms show the sacral cornua and caudal epidural space before (**A**) and after (**B**) injection of local anesthetic. The injection of local anesthetic distributes throughout the caudal epidural space and tents the sacrococcygeal ligament.

Head and Neck Blocks

CHAPTER 55

MENTAL NERVE BLOCK

The mental nerve is a branch of the inferior alveolar nerve from the third division of the trigeminal nerve. The inferior alveolar nerve enters the mandibular foramen to travel within the mandibular canal and form the mental nerve. At its exit from the mental foramen, the mental nerve is divided into several branches.[1] The mental nerve emerges from the mental foramen to supply the chin, lower lip, and teeth. The mental nerve can provide innervation to the lower incisors.[2]

The mental foramen lies about halfway between the upper and lower borders of the mandible, although the position of the foramen relative to the mandible varies with age.[3,4] Elderly patients who are edentulous will have decay of the alveolar ridge. This brings the mental foramen closer to the upper border of the mandible. A severely resorbed alveolar ridge can make identification of the mental foramen difficult.

Suggested Technique

Ultrasound imaging can establish foramen location and morphology for optimal approach. With proper needle positioning within the canal, more extensive block can result.

The mental foramen typically has posterior or right-angled inclination.[5] When the nerve emerges at right angles, it is funnel shaped. The longest diameter of the mental foramen is about 3 mm.[6] The presence of multiple mental foramina is rare, being observed in about 2% of cases.[3-5,7]

For this block, the operator stands at the head of the bed and faces the feet of the patient. The block needle is advanced well into the mental canal (~6 mm) for successful block and to achieve anesthesia of the lower incisors. For this, 1- to 2-mL injection of local anesthetic is required. The block needle passes through the platysma and depressor anguli oris muscles on the approach to the canal. Care is taken not to puncture the facial artery, which usually lies on the posterior side of the foramen.

Clinical Pearls

- Advance the block needle 6 mm into the mental canal for successful block.
- Local anesthetic injected within the mental foramen will track centrally along the inferior alveolar nerve within the mandibular canal.
- Use a 25-gauge 38-mm needle for placement in the mental canal.
- Facial hair can make imaging for mental canal block challenging.
- The facial artery and vein lie close to the mental foramen.

References

1. Hu KS, Yun HS, Hur MS, et al. Branching patterns and intraosseous course of the mental nerve. *J Oral Maxillofac Surg.* 2007;65:2288-2294.
2. Pogrel MA, Smith R, Ahani R. Innervation of the mandibular incisors by the mental nerve. *J Oral Maxillofac Surg.* 1997; 55:961-963.
3. Vayvada H, Demirdover C, Yilmaz M, Barutcu A. An anatomic variation of the mental nerve and foramina: a case report. *Clin Anat.* 2006;19:700-701.
4. Oktem H, Oktem F, Sanli E, et al. An anatomic variation of mental nerve. *Plast Reconstr Aesthet Surg.* 2008;61:1408-1409.
5. Kieser J, Kuzmanovic D, Payne A, et al. Patterns of emergence of the human mental nerve. *Arch Oral Biol.* 2002;47:743-747.
6. Song WC, Kim SH, Paik DJ, et al. Location of the infraorbital and mental foramen with reference to the soft-tissue landmarks. *Plast Reconstr Surg.* 2007;120:1343-1347.
7. Agthong S, Huanmanop T, Chentanez V. Anatomical variations of the supraorbital, infraorbital, and mental foramina related to gender and side. *J Oral Maxillofac Surg.* 2005;63:800-804.

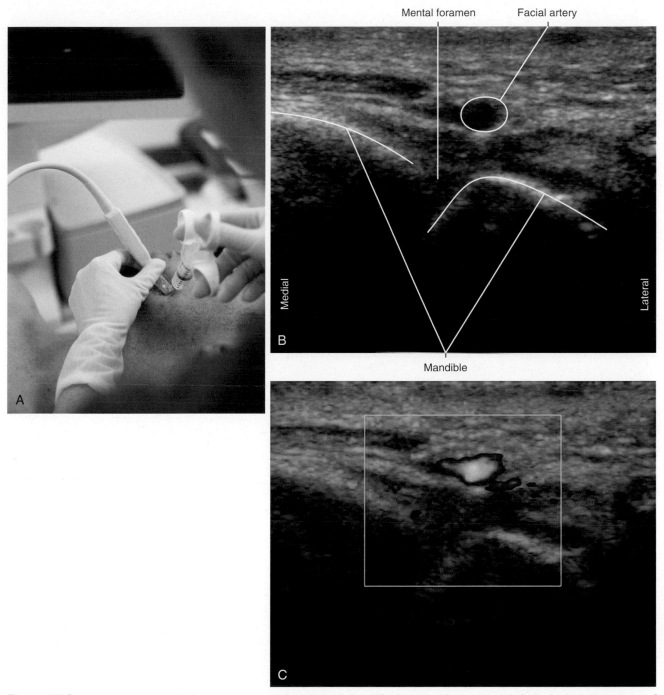

Figure 55-1. External photograph showing an approach to mental nerve block. An in-plane approach from the posterior aspect of the mandible is shown (**A**). The corresponding sonogram of the mental foramen is shown (**B**). Power Doppler verifies the presence of a blood vessel lying over the foramen (**C**).

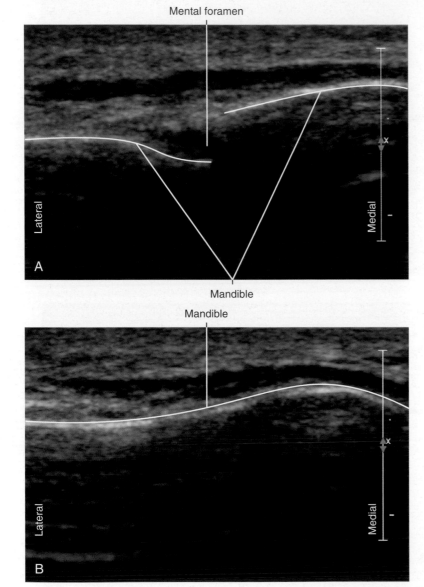

Mental foramen

Lateral

Medial

x

A

Mandible

Mandible

Lateral

Medial

x

B

Figure 55-2. Ultrasound image of the mental foramen (**A**) contrasted with the smooth bony contour of the mandible (**B**).

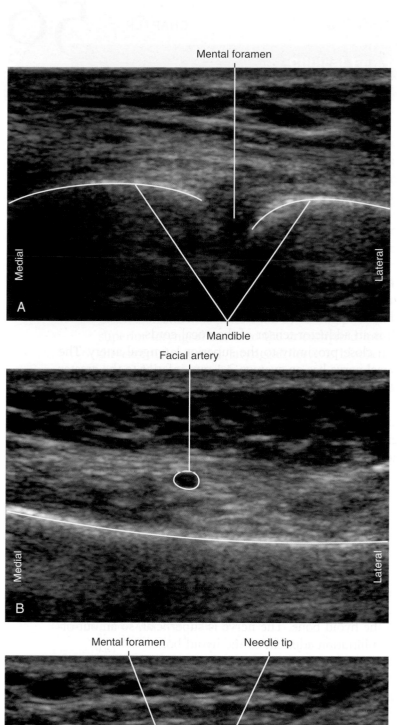

Mental foramen

Medial

Lateral

A

Mandible

Facial artery

Medial

Lateral

B

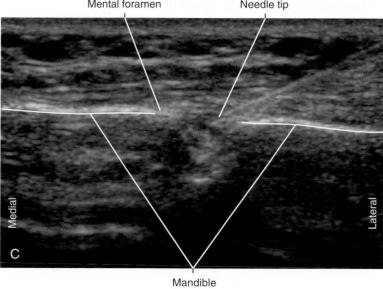

Mental foramen   Needle tip

Medial

Lateral

C

Mandible

Figure 55-3. Image sequence showing mental nerve block in the mental foramen. The mental foramen is first identified and the angle of approach planned (**A**). The facial artery is identified posterior to the mental foramen (**B**). The block needle is placed within the mental foramen for injection of local anesthetic (**C**).

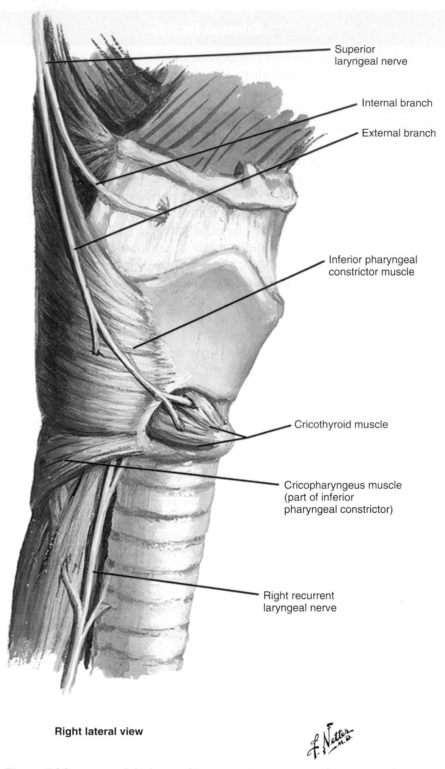

Right lateral view

Figure 56-1. Nerves of the larynx. (From netterimages.com, with permission.)

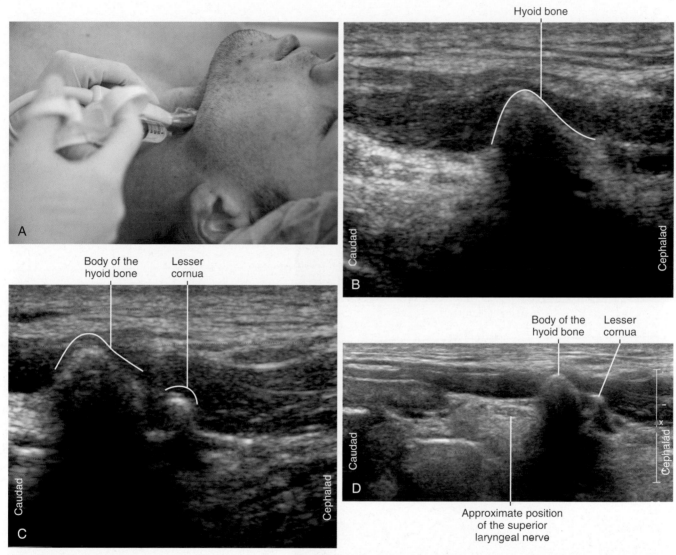

Figure 56-2. External photograph showing an approach to superior laryngeal nerve block with ultrasound imaging. An out-of-plane approach from the lateral aspect of the neck is shown (**A**). Corresponding sonograms for a short-axis view of the hyoid bone (**B**), at the level of the lesser cornua (**C**), and view with a broad linear probe (**D**). The hyoid bone can give a triangular acoustic shadow when viewed in short axis that can help identify its location. The hyoid bone has two horns, the lesser (superior) cornua and the greater (inferior) cornua. The superior cornua of the hyoid bone is highly echogenic. Despite its name, the greater (longer) horn of the hyoid bone is difficult to image because the hyoid bone narrows substantially in the posterior direction.

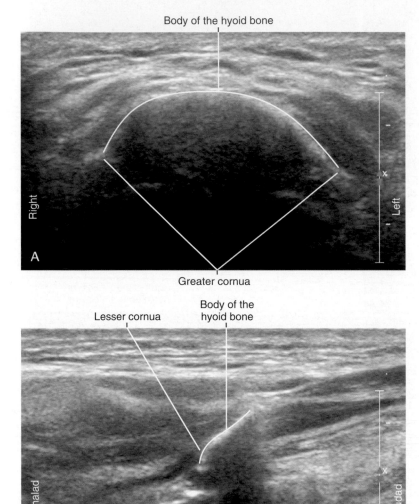

Body of the hyoid bone

Right

Left

A

Greater cornua

Lesser cornua

Body of the hyoid bone

Cephalad

Caudad

B

Figure 56-3. Long-axis view of the hyoid bone (**A**) shown with a sloping short-axis view of the lesser cornua (**B**). The hyoid is a small U-shaped bone as seen in this long-axis view. The internal branch of the superior laryngeal nerve lies immediately inferior and deep to the greater cornua of the hyoid bone.

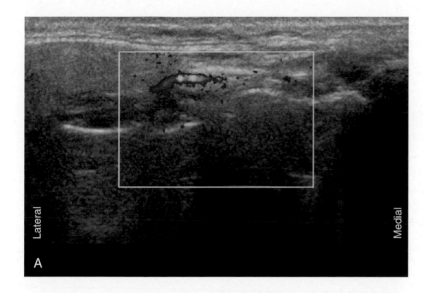

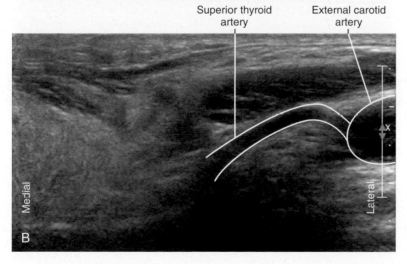

Figure 56-4. Power Doppler imaging of the superior laryngeal artery as it descends into the larynx (**A**). The superior laryngeal nerve lies superior to the superior laryngeal artery. Sonogram showing the origin of the superior thyroid artery from the external carotid (**B**). The superior thyroid artery is the first branch of the external carotid artery. It gives rise to the superior laryngeal artery.

CHAPTER 57

GREAT AURICULAR NERVE BLOCK

The great auricular nerve (GAN) is the largest branch of the superficial cervical plexus (see Chapter 58, Fig. 58-1). It provides cutaneous innervation to the periauricular region. The GAN wraps around the posterior border of the sternocleidomastoid muscle (SCM) and then courses superiorly and anteriorly, dividing into anterior and posterior branches.[1] Because of its superficial location, the GAN can be damaged during surgical procedures in the neck.[2] The nerves of the superficial cervical plexus lie deep to the platysma when first emerging from the plexus, but superficial to the prevertebral fascia.

The GAN lies superficial to the lateral border of the SCM and can be traced to the preauricular area or back to the superficial cervical plexus. The lesser occipital nerve has similar anatomy, except that it can be followed behind the ear.

Suggested Technique

The GAN has a characteristic monofascicular or bifascicular appearance on ultrasound scans where it courses over the SCM. The GAN flattens in shape slightly as it lies over the SCM. The nerve becomes difficult to image at the lateral corner of the SCM. This point is about the level of the cricoid cartilage. Isolated GAN blocks are possible, but its large size and characteristic ultrasound appearance make the GAN a convenient way of identifying the position of the remainder of the superficial cervical plexus.

Because the GAN is very superficial, an out-of-plane approach to GAN block is usually used with the nerve viewed in short axis. The GAN lies near the external jugular vein, so vascular puncture and minor bleeding is possible.

Clinical Pearls

- The GAN consists of contributions from the second and third cervical nerves. The GAN divides into anterior and posterior branches.
- The GAN can have a small mastoid branch that lies close to the lesser occipital nerve (observed in 16 of 24 specimens).[3]
- Dominance patterns of cutaneous innervation of the external ear has been examined.[4] Most patterns are either lesser occipital or great auricular dominant.

References

1. Ginsberg LE, Eicher SA. Great auricular nerve: anatomy and imaging in a case of perineural tumor spread. *AJNR Am J Neuroradiol.* 2000;21:568-571.
2. Nusair YM, Dickenson AJ. Great auricular causalgia: an unusual complication of excision of the submandibular gland. *Br J Oral Maxillofac Surg.* 2003;41:334-335.
3. Tubbs RS, Salter EG, Wellons JC, et al. Landmarks for the identification of the cutaneous nerves of the occiput and nuchal regions. *Clin Anat.* 2007;20:235-238.
4. Pantaloni M, Sullivan P. Relevance of the lesser occipital nerve in facial rejuvenation surgery. *Plast Reconstr Surg.* 2000; 105:2594-2599.

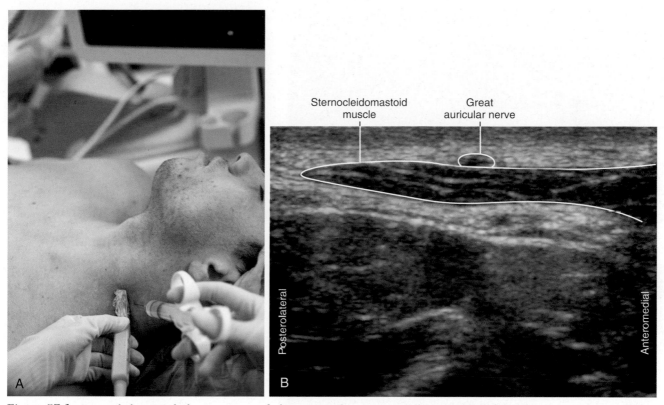

Figure 57-1. External photograph showing an out-of-plane approach to great auricular nerve block (**A**). The corresponding sonogram is shown before needle placement (**B**).

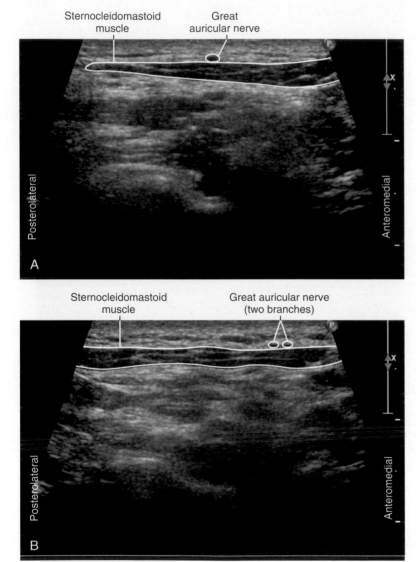

Figure 57-2. Short-axis view of the great auricular nerve near the posterolateral border of the sternocleidomastoid muscle (**A**). The great auricular nerve divides into anterior and posterior branches (**B**).

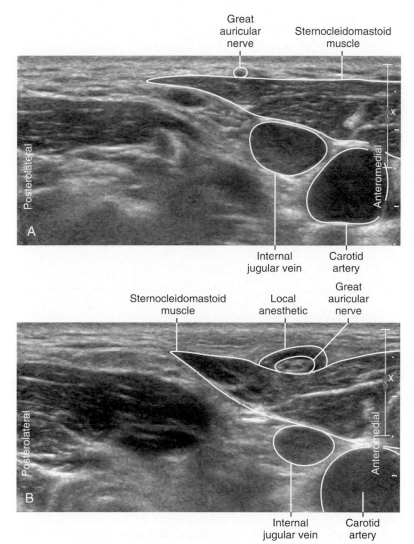

Figure 57-3. Short-axis view of the great auricular nerve before (**A**) and after (**B**) injection of local anesthetic. Local anesthetic is seen to distribute around the nerve.

CHAPTER 58

SUPERFICIAL CERVICAL PLEXUS BLOCK

The superficial cervical plexus (SCP) derives from the ventral rami of C2, C3, and C4. Its branches primarily consist of the lesser occipital, great auricular, transverse cervical, and supraclavicular nerves. These nerves innervate the skin of the neck and shoulder. The nerves converge at the lateral border of the sternocleidomastoid muscle at the level of the cricoid cartilage. The great auricular nerve is the largest and most easily identifiable nerve of the superficial cervical plexus. This nerve can be used to estimate the position of the remainder of the superficial cervical plexus. Indications for superficial cervical plexus block include carotid endarterectomy and clavicle surgery.[1] Ultrasound can be used to guide a variety of cervical plexus blocks.[2,3]

Suggested Technique

The SCP can be blocked by using a medial to lateral in-plane approach. Using this approach, the needle tip is positioned through the tapering lateral edge of the sternocleidomastoid muscle at the level of the cricoid cartilage. The needle tip should be deep to the platysma and sternocleidomastoid muscle but superficial to the prevertebral fascia that covers the brachial plexus, scalene muscles, and phrenic nerve. Local anesthetic distributes deep to the undersurface of the sternocleidomastoid muscle. This trans-sternocleidomastoid approach to superficial cervical plexus block is used to place the needle tip in the correct layer, which is deep to the subcutaneous tissue.[4]

If the great auricular nerve is identified, the block can be performed caudal to where this nerve crosses over the sternocleidomastoid. Because the block is very superficial, the tapering lateral edge of the sternocleidomastoid can be imaged at the edge of the screen near the approaching needle. A 25-gauge, 1.5-inch hypodermic needle on extension tubing or control syringe can be used for the block.

Similar to the brachial plexus, the cervical plexus emerges between the anterior and middle scalene muscles.[5] If interscalene brachial plexus block is performed, injection as the needle is pulled back will anesthetize the SCP.

Because the phrenic nerve separates from the C5 ventral ramus at the level of the cricoid cartilage, it can serve as a landmark for the location of the SCP. However, unlike the phrenic nerve, the SCP lies superficial to the prevertebral fascia. Phrenic nerve blocks can occur during cervical plexus blocks.[6]

Intravascular injection is one of the most frequent complications of cervical plexus block.[7] This may relate to the proximity of the external jugular vein.

Clinical Pearls

- One classic approach to cervical plexus block in the interscalene groove is to inject deep to the prevertebral fascia at the superior margin of the thyroid cartilage, which approximates C4.[5] With this approach, the nerves are blocked before they pierce the prevertebral fascia.
- SCP blocks can be assessed from the clavicle to behind the ear along the posterolateral border of the sternocleidomastoid muscle.

References

1. Choi DS, Atchabahian A, Brown AR. Cervical plexus block provides postoperative analgesia after clavicle surgery. *Anesth Analg.* 2005;100:1542-1543.
2. Sandeman DJ, Griffiths MJ, Lennox AF. Ultrasound guided deep cervical plexus block. *Anaesth Intens Care.* 2006;34:240-244.
3. Roessel T, Wiessner D, Heller AR, et al. High-resolution ultrasound-guided high interscalene plexus block for carotid endarterectomy. *Reg Anesth Pain Med.* 2007;32:247-253.
4. Pandit JJ, Dutta D, Morris JF. Spread of injectate with superficial cervical plexus block in humans: an anatomical study. *Br J Anaesth.* 2003;91:733-735.
5. Winnie AP, Ramamurthy S, Durrani Z, Radonjic R. Interscalene cervical plexus block: a single-injection technic. *Anesth Analg.* 1975;54:370-375.
6. Emery G, Handley G, Davies MJ, Mooney PH. Incidence of phrenic nerve block and hypercapnia in patients undergoing carotid endarterectomy under cervical plexus block. *Anaesth Intens Care.* 1998;26:377-381.
7. Davies MJ, Silbert BS, Scott DA, et al. Superficial and deep cervical plexus block for carotid artery surgery: a prospective study of 1000 blocks. *Reg Anesth.* 1997;22:442-446.

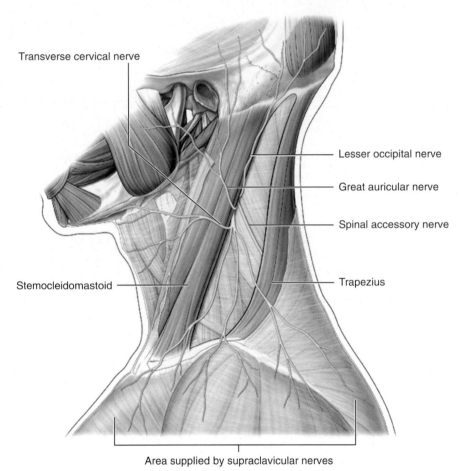

Transverse cervical nerve

Lesser occipital nerve

Great auricular nerve

Spinal accessory nerve

Sternocleidomastoid

Trapezius

Area supplied by supraclavicular nerves

Figure 58-1. The cutaneous branches of the cervical plexus. The spinal part of the accessory nerve that supplies the trapezius is also shown as it crosses the posterior triangle. Note that the interval between the upper attachments of sternocleidomastoid and trapezius is not normally as extensive as shown here. (From Standring S. *Gray's Anatomy*, 40th ed. Philadelphia: Elsevier; 2009. Figure 28.1.)

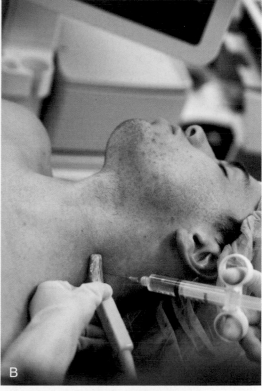

Figure 58-2. External photographs showing approaches to superficial cervical plexus block. An in-plane approach from medial to lateral is shown (**A**). An out-of-plane approach is shown (**B**).

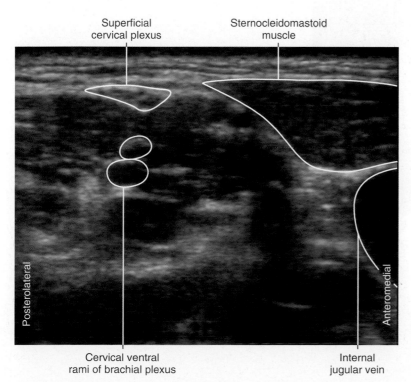

Superficial
cervical plexus

Sternocleidomastoid
muscle

Posterolateral

Anteromedial

Cervical ventral
rami of brachial plexus

Internal
jugular vein

Figure 58-3. Short-axis view of the superficial cervical plexus. The plexus is seen at the tapering lateral edge of the sternocleidomastoid muscle that forms an acute angle. This corner of the muscle is where superficial cervical plexus block is performed.

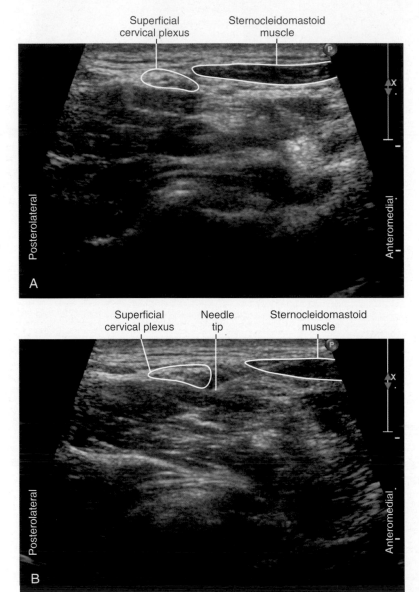

Figure 58-4. Image sequence showing superficial plexus block. An in-plane approach is demonstrated where the needle tip is placed under the superficial cervical plexus (**A**). After injection, local anesthetic is distributed around the nerves (**B**).

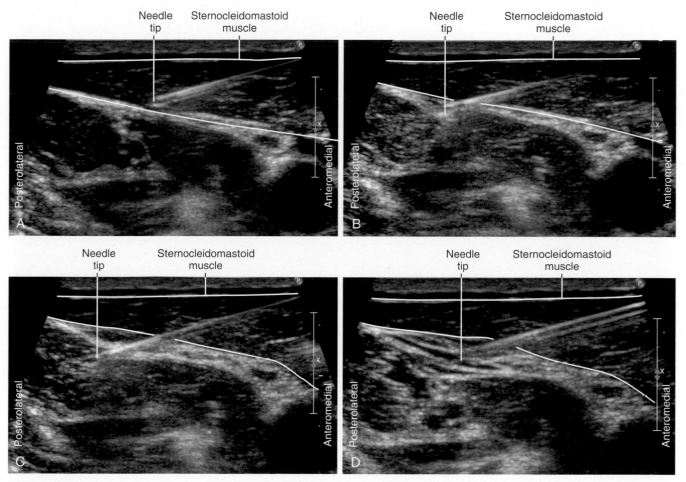

Figure 58-5. When the superficial cervical plexus is difficult to identify, local anesthetic can be injected under the posterolateral edge of the sternocleidomastoid muscle. This image sequence shows the process of needle placement and injection (**A** through **D**). Care must be taken to avoid the phrenic nerve, spinal accessory nerve, and brachial plexus.

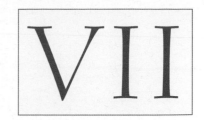

Safety Issues

CHAPTER 59

ADVERSE EVENTS

It is important to be able to prevent and recognize adverse events that can occur during ultrasound-guided regional blocks. Ultrasound-guided regional anesthesia has demonstrated efficacy, and now safety issues require careful examination. Because adverse events are uncommon, these issues will take time to assess within the broad spectrum of clinical practice. Although most evidence would suggest that ultrasound guidance improves safety, there are important limitations to the technology.[1] Education and training play major roles in safety of ultrasound-guided interventions. Tissue-equivalent phantoms that simulate ultrasound-guided interventions are excellent tools to demonstrate needle tip visibility and other training issues.

Clinical Pearls

- Ultrasound imaging can detect intravascular and intraneural injections.
- Ultrasound has a limited ability to ascertain nerve borders and individual nerve fascicles.
- Training phantoms need to be developed that reflect the complexity of clinical imaging.

Reference

1. Nolsoe C, Nielsen L, Torp-Pedersen S, Holm HH. Major complications and deaths due to interventional ultrasonography: a review of 8000 cases. *J Clin Ultrasound.* 1990;18:179-184.

CHAPTER 60

INTRAVASCULAR INJECTIONS

Ultrasound guidance for regional blocks appears to reduce but not eliminate the vascular puncture risk. This is similar to what has been reported for ultrasound guidance for other interventions.[1]

Small-volume test injections (0.5-1 mL) are useful for detecting intravascular injections.[2] If the injection is not visualized, it should be stopped immediately. It is best to presume intravascular injection or some other adverse event.

Systemic toxicity of local anesthetics is probably reduced with ultrasound guidance for several reasons. First, evidence suggests that regional blocks can be performed with lower volumes of local anesthetic. Second, the chance of vascular puncture by the needle tip is less. Third, it is possible to recognize intravascular injection. This detection occurs dynamically on-line (effectively in real-time at frame rates >30 frames per second).

Despite this favorable safety profile, intravascular injection with systemic toxicity has been reported with ultrasound guidance.[3,4] Another concern is that probe compression may prevent detection of intravenous injection by collapsing the vein after puncture.[5] It is difficult to assess the incidence of these problems from case reports, but these events are likely uncommon and primarily relate to limitations in needle tip visibility. Vascular puncture rates reported from clinical studies of ultrasound-guided regional blocks are listed in Table 60-1.[6-11]

TABLE 60-1 Vascular Puncture Rates Reported From Clinical Studies of Ultrasound-Guided Regional Blocks

BLOCK	ULTRASOUND	CONTROL	REFERENCE
Supraclavicular	1 in 40 (2.5%)	None	Chan et al[6] (2003)
Infraclavicular	8 in 1146 (0.7%)	None	Sandhu et al[7] (2006)
Axillary	0 in 146 (0%)	0 in 72 (0%)	Chan et al[8] (2007)
Femoral	0 in 20 (0%)	3 in 20 (15%)	Marhofer et al[10] (1997)
Femoral	0 in 20 (0%)	4 in 40 (10%)	Marhofer et al[9] (1998)
Multiple	3 in 124 (2.4%)	12 in 124 (9.7%)	Orebaugh et al[11] (2007)

References

1. Randolph AG, Cook DJ, Gonzales CA, Pribble CG. Ultrasound guidance for placement of central venous catheters: a meta-analysis of the literature. *Crit Care Med.* 1996;24:2053-2058.
2. VadeBoncouer TR, Weinberg GL, Oswald S, Angelov F. Early detection of intravascular injection during ultrasound-guided supraclavicular brachial plexus block. *Reg Anesth Pain Med.* 2008;33:278-279.
3. Loubert C, Williams SR, Hélie F, Arcand G. Complication during ultrasound-guided regional block: accidental intravascular injection of local anesthetic. *Anesthesiology.* 2008;108:759-760.
4. Zetlaoui PJ, Labbe JP, Benhamou D. Ultrasound guidance for axillary plexus block does not prevent intravascular injection. *Anesthesiology.* 2008;108:761.
5. Robards C, Clendenen S, Greengrass R. Intravascular injection during ultrasound-guided axillary block: negative aspiration can be misleading. *Anesth Analg.* 2008;107:1754-1755.
6. Chan VW, Perlas A, Rawson R, Odukoya O. Ultrasound-guided supraclavicular brachial plexus block. *Anesth Analg.* 2003;97:1514-1517.
7. Sandhu NS, Manne JS, Medabalmi PK, Capan LM. Sonographically guided infraclavicular brachial plexus block in adults: a retrospective analysis of 1146 cases. *J Ultrasound Med.* 2006;25:1555-1561.
8. Chan VW, Perlas A, McCartney CJ, et al. Ultrasound guidance improves success rate of axillary brachial plexus block. *Can J Anaesth.* 2007;54:176-182.
9. Marhofer P, Schrogendorfer K, Wallner T, et al. Ultrasonographic guidance reduces the amount of local anesthetic for 3-in-1 blocks. *Reg Anesth Pain Med.* 1998;23:584-588.
10. Marhofer P, Schrögendorfer K, Koinig H, et al. Ultrasonographic guidance improves sensory block and onset time of three-in-one blocks. *Anesth Analg.* 1997;85:854-857.
11. Orebaugh SL, Williams BA, Kentor ML. Ultrasound guidance with nerve stimulation reduces the time necessary for resident peripheral nerve blockade. *Reg Anesth Pain Med.* 32:448-454, 2007.

Axillary
artery

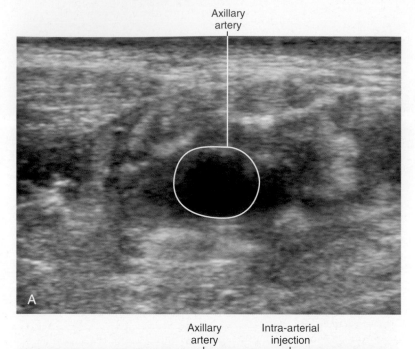

Axillary   Intra-arterial
artery   injection

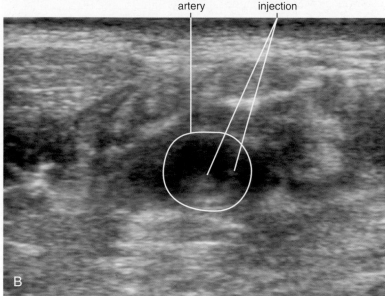

Figure 60-1. Ultrasound detection of intra-arterial injection of local anesthetic. The axillary artery is shown in short-axis view before (**A**) and after (**B**) injection of local anesthetic for out-of-plane axillary block.

CHAPTER 61

INTRANEURAL INJECTIONS

Safety issues for ultrasound in regional anesthesia practice have been raised by several authors.[1,2] Tremendous controversy and debate surround this field, particularly in regard to the subject of intraneural injection.

A large number of seemingly innocuous intraneural injections imaged with ultrasound have now been reported.[1,3,4] In these cases, although nerve expansion from injection was reported, no loss of nerve border integrity was detected. All these intraneural injections were believed to be low pressure. Most of these harmless intraneural injections have been detected by retrospective review of ultrasound recordings of blocks and were not recognized on-line in real time. All these intraneural injections were in nerves with high collagen content and polyfascicular architecture. There have been no reported cases of intraneural injections in monofascicular nerves, which would more likely result in functional damage.

Peripheral nerves normally have substantial regenerative capacity. However, in a number of clinical conditions, this capacity is limited (e.g., neuropathy from diabetes, alcoholism).

We have yet to establish the sonographic signs of intraneural injections that produce functional damage. To date, there has been only one published report of sonographic nerve imaging following nerve injury resulting from needle injection.[5] Sonography cannot distinguish between subepineurial and subperineurial needle tip placement. Subperineurial injection is thought to be most harmful.[6]

Intraneural injections have been dichotomized into high-pressure and low-pressure types.[7,8] The low-pressure type has not been associated with injury and may be common in clinical practice. Collateral damage may be the mechanism of adjacent fiber injury after high-pressure injection (nerve blast injury from explosion with surrounding nerve fascicles damaged).

Ultrasound may be able to identify some factors that influence the chance of nerve injury during regional anesthetics. Nerve echotexture may play an important role in perioperative nerve injuries. Polyfascicular nerves contain more protective connective tissue than monofascicular nerves. The outcomes after monofascicular nerve injuries are probably worse than after polyfascicular injuries.[9]

Nerves are usually mobile and distensible structures. However, if nerve fascicles become trapped on both sides of the advancing needle, paresthesia often occurs as the needle crosses into or even through the nerve. The complex architecture of peripheral nerves in regard to somatotopic orientation of motor and sensory fibers may account for the variability in mechanically and electrically evoked responses. Ultrasound also can identify proximity to underlying structures that are an unyielding surface. Nerve blocks performed near bone have been associated with a high incidence of nerve dysfunction.[10]

Nerve shape also may play a role in nerve injury. Round nerves are less likely to be impaled because the needle moves to the side during needle advancement. Injection within a nerve can be similar to blowing up a deflated balloon; the nerve will become more round with injection. Any change in nerve shape or increase in cross-sectional area during injection should be considered serious. The injection should be halted because there is no benefit from further injection inside the nerve, and there is potential harm. Nerve fascicles themselves are always round, and therefore monofascicular nerves are normally round.

By identifying ultrasound characteristics of needle-induced nerve injury, we can potentially reduce the incidence of neurologic complications after regional block. New strategies for ultrasound block techniques can be developed that minimize future risks.

Clinical Pearls

- Traumatic nerve lesions are characterized by nerve enlargement, nerve hyperemia, loss of fascicular discrimination, swelling proximal to the injured segment, and change in nerve caliber.
- Intraneural needle tip placement is often only recognized after injection (and even then, by retrospective review of recorded images rather than on-line).
- Factors that influence regenerative capacity of peripheral nerves include diabetes, preexisting neuropathy, age, and others.
- Adverse symptoms have been reported after intentional intraneural injection of local anesthetics.[11]
- Adverse neurologic outcome related to needle injection has been reported without sonographic evidence of intraneural injection.[12]

References

1. Schafhalter-Zoppoth I, Zeitz ID, Gray AT. Inadvertent femoral nerve impalement and intraneural injection visualized by ultrasound. *Anesth Analg.* 2004;99:627-628.
2. Chan VW, Brull R, McCartney CJ, et al. An ultrasonographic and histological study of intraneural injection and electrical stimulation in pigs. *Anesth Analg.* 2007;104:1281-1284.
3. Bigeleisen PE. Nerve puncture and apparent intraneural injection during ultrasound-guided axillary block does not invariably result in neurologic injury. *Anesthesiology.* 2006;105:779-783.
4. Russon K, Blanco R. Accidental intraneural injection into the musculocutaneous nerve visualized with ultrasound. *Anesth Analg.* 105:1504-1505, 2007.
5. Graif M, Seton A, Nerubai J, et al. Sciatic nerve: sonographic evaluation and anatomic-pathologic considerations. *Radiology.* 1991;181:405-408.
6. Gentili F, Hudson A, Kline DG, Hunter D. Peripheral nerve injection injury: an experimental study. *Neurosurgery.* 1979;4:244-253.
7. Selander D, Sjostrand J. Longitudinal spread of intraneurally injected local anesthetics: an experimental study of the initial neural distribution following intraneural injections. *Acta Anaesthesiol Scand.* 1978;22:622-634.
8. Hadzic A, Dilberovic F, Shah S, et al. Combination of intraneural injection and high injection pressure leads to fascicular injury and neurologic deficits in dogs. *Reg Anesth Pain Med.* 2004;29:417-423.
9. Sunderland S. The anatomy and physiology of nerve injury. *Muscle Nerve.* 1990;13:771-784.
10. Lofstrom B, Wennberg A, Wien L. Late disturbances in nerve function after block with local anaesthetic agents: an electroneurographic study. *Acta Anaesthesiol Scand.* 1966;10:111-122.
11. Lee J, Lee YS. Percutaneous chemical nerve block with ultrasound-guided intraneural injection. *Eur Radiol.* 2008;18:1506-1512.
12. Koff MD, Cohen JA, McIntyre JJ, et al. Severe brachial plexopathy after an ultrasound-guided single-injection nerve block for total shoulder arthroplasty in a patient with multiple sclerosis. *Anesthesiology.* 2008;108:325-328.

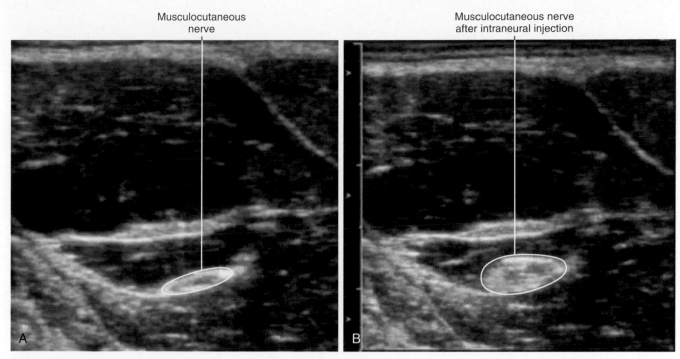

Musculocutaneous
nerve

Musculocutaneous nerve
after intraneural injection

Figure 61-1. Short-axis view of an intraneural injection during musculocutaneous nerve block in the axilla. Before injection (**A**) and after injection (**B**). This event was recognized afterward by retrospective review of the block recording.

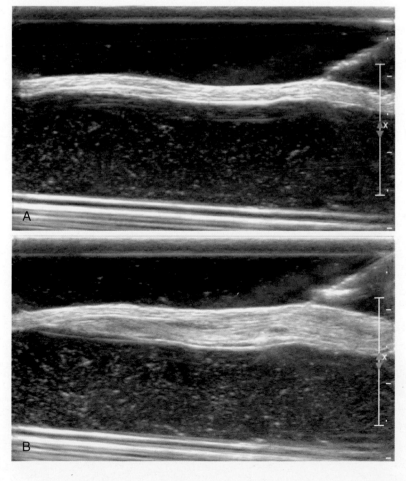

Figure 61-2. Simulated intraneural injection in an excised ex vivo specimen before (**A**) and after (**B**) injection. Long-axis view of a peripheral nerve demonstrating fusiform enlargement after intraneural injection with in-plane approach of the needle. Change in the nerve caliber occurs in the region of the injection.

CHAPTER 62

PNEUMOTHORAX AND OTHER CHEST PATHOLOGY

Ultrasound imaging can prevent and diagnose pneumothorax. Chest sonography is therefore an essential skill for those performing regional blocks. Regional anesthesia is the leading cause of pneumothorax during anesthesia, and twice as likely as the next leading cause.[1] This is particularly surprisingly given that line placement is another potential cause of perioperative pneumothorax.

The incidence of pneumothorax after traditional supraclavicular block has been reported to be as high as 0.5% to 6%.[2] This high incidence has led to concern that supraclavicular blocks should not be performed on outpatients. Pneumothorax after ultrasound-guided regional block has now been reported.[3]

Several risk factors for pneumothorax and chest tube placement have been identified in patients undergoing interventional procedures.[4] These include the needle traversing aerated lung or a lung fissure, lung hyperinflation from chronic obstructive lung disease, and positive-pressure ventilation.

Surprisingly, even when the needle traverses aerated lung, the pneumothorax risk is only about 50%, probably because in many cases, the lung heals on its own. In some studies, chronic obstructive lung disease doubled the risk for pneumothorax, with an even greater risk for chest tube placement. This risk is thought to be related to lung hyperinflation and the fragile composition of the lung.

Because of the marked acoustic impedance mismatch with soft tissue, the pleura generates a brighter echo than the surface of the first rib. Comet-tail artifact can be observed deep to strongly reflecting structures, such as the lung.[5,6] The comet-tail artifact usually manifests as dense, continuous echoes.

Lung sliding is the to-and-fro movement of the lung caused by respiration. Because most of the translational motion of ventilated lung is generated from descent of the diaphragm, lung sliding is smallest at the apex and maximal at the base. Therefore, lung sliding can be difficult to appreciate during supraclavicular views of the brachial plexus. In this location, the first rib and pleura are best distinguished by the absorption of ultrasound by the bone and comet-tail artifact that arises from the pleural line. The presence of lung sliding or comet-tail artifact rules out pneumothorax.[7,8]

Clinical Pearls

- Postinterventional sonograms are often obtained to rule out pneumothorax.[9]
- Sonography can be used to reveal the lung point, which is the border between aerated lung and pneumothorax.

References

1. Cheney FW, Posner KL, Caplan RA. Adverse respiratory events infrequently leading to malpractice suits: a closed claims analysis. *Anesthesiology*. 1991;75:932-939.
2. Brown DL, Cahill DR, Bridenbaugh LD. Supraclavicular nerve block: anatomic analysis of a method to prevent pneumothorax. *Anesth Analg*. 1993;76:530-534.
3. Bryan NA, Swenson JD, Greis PE, Burks RT. Indwelling interscalene catheter use in an outpatient setting for shoulder surgery: technique, efficacy, and complications. *J Shoulder Elbow Surg*. 2007;16:388-395.
4. Cox JE, Chiles C, McManus CM, et al. Transthoracic needle aspiration biopsy: variables that affect risk of pneumothorax. *Radiology*. 1999;212:165-168.
5. Ziskin MC, Thickman DI, Goldenberg NJ, et al. The comet tail artifact. *J Ultrasound Med*. 1982;1:1-7.
6. Thickman DI, Ziskin MC, Goldenberg NJ, Linder BE. Clinical manifestations of the comet tail artifact. *J Ultrasound Med*. 1983;2:225-230.
7. Lichtenstein DA, Menu Y. A bedside ultrasound sign ruling out pneumothorax in the critically ill: lung sliding. *Chest*. 1995;108:1345-1348.
8. Lichtenstein D, Meziere G, Biderman P, Gepner A. The comet-tail artifact: an ultrasound sign ruling out pneumothorax. *Intensive Care Med*. 1999;25:383-388.
9. Reissig A, Kroegel C. Accuracy of transthoracic sonography in excluding post-interventional pneumothorax and hydropneumothorax: comparison to chest radiography. *Eur J Radiol*. 2005;53:463-470.

Ribs

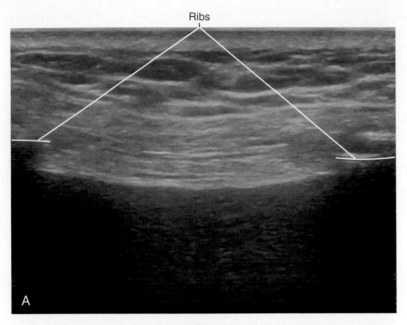

A

Ribs

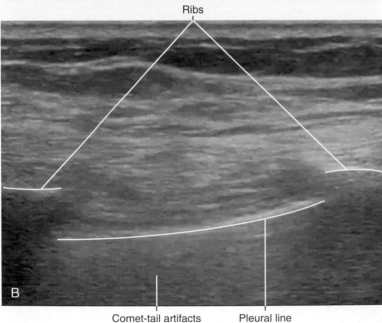

B

Comet-tail artifacts   Pleural line

Figure 62-1. Loss of the comet-tail artifact from the pleural line (**A**). Sonogram of the control lung is shown for comparison (**B**). In this example, the loss of the comet-tail artifact was from massive hydrothorax.

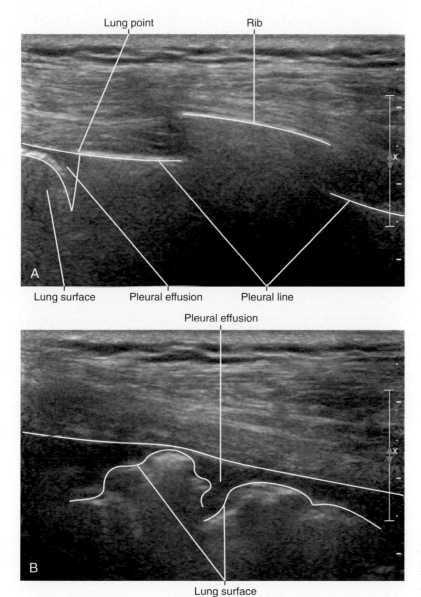

Figure 62-2. Sonography can be used to reveal the lung point, which is the border between aerated and nonaerated lung (**A**). In this example, the cause of formation of the lung point was pleural effusion (**B**).

SELF-ASSESSMENT QUESTIONS: TEXT

1. Why do peripheral nerves often appear more echogenic after injection of anechoic local anesthetic?
   A. The connective tissue content of the nerves has increased.
   B. Nonattenuating fluid has been injected into an attenuating sound field.
   C. The number of fascicles has increased.
   D. Local anesthetic has entered the nerve and increased reflection.

2. Which of the following statements regarding peripheral nerve anatomy is most correct?
   A. Polyfascicular nerves have a low connective tissue content compared with monofascicular nerves.
   B. The cervical ventral rami have a high connective tissue content.
   C. The number of fascicles and the connective tissue content of peripheral nerves are directly related.
   D. Nerve fascicles are made exclusively of connective tissue.

3. Which of the following is most accurate?
   A. Ultrasound frequencies of 10 MHz or higher are necessary to distinguish peripheral nerves from tendons based on echotexture alone.
   B. Peripheral nerves can only be imaged with ultrasound frequencies of 10 MHz or higher.
   C. Peripheral nerves can only be imaged with ultrasound frequencies of 20 MHz or higher.
   D. Peripheral nerves and tendons cannot be distinguished with ultrasound imaging.

4. Which of the following statements regarding probe compression is most correct?
   A. Nerves do not move in response to probe compression.
   B. Arteries cannot be compressed by the ultrasound probe.
   C. Veins are easier to compress than arteries.
   D. Nerves are easily compressed by the ultrasound probe.

5. What term describes the fact that the received echoes from peripheral nerves vary with the angle of insonation?
   A. Acoustic emission
   B. Anisotropy
   C. Power Doppler imaging
   D. None of the above

6. Which of the following statements is most accurate?
   A. Nerves are more anisotropic than tendons.
   B. The anisotropy of peripheral nerves is thought related to their myelin content rather than their collagen content.
   C. The amplitude of the received echoes from peripheral nerves is usually largest when the sound beam is perpendicular to the nerve.
   D. Nerves and tendons do not exhibit anisotropy.

7. Which of the following influences needle tip visibility? (Select all that apply.)
   A. The angle of insonation
   B. The gauge of the needle
   C. The bevel orientation
   D. The bevel angle

8. Which of following is associated with comet-tail artifact?
   A. First rib
   B. Pneumothorax
   C. Normal pleura
   D. Brachial plexus

9. Select the best answer.
   A. Bone is a strong absorber of sound waves.
   B. Pleura is a strong reflector of sound waves.
   C. Both of the above statements are true.

10. Which of the following statements regarding interscalene block is true?
    A. The phrenic nerve lies medial to the brachial plexus within the middle scalene muscle.
    B. The phrenic nerve crosses over the anterior scalene muscle medial to the brachial plexus.
    C. The dorsal scapular nerve is often seen within the anterior scalene muscle.
    D. The spinal accessory nerve arises from the brachial plexus.

11. Which of the following statements regarding the first rib and pleura is true?
    A. Only the first rib produces comet-tail artifact.
    B. Comet-tail artifact signifies the presence of pneumothorax.
    C. The pleura produces a bright reflection and comet-tail artifact.
    D. The first rib does not produce reflection of sound waves.

12. What is the most common anatomic variation in the interscalene region?
    A. Cervical rib
    B. Cervical ventral rami that pass over or through the anterior scalene muscle
    C. Phrenic nerve passing through the middle scalene muscle
    D. Phrenic nerve passing through the subclavian artery

13. The phrenic nerve lies on which muscle in the neck?

14. The cords of the brachial plexus are named with respect to what structure?

15. What branches leave the brachial plexus sheath under the pectoralis minor at the coracoid process?

16. At the level of an axillary block, the musculocutaneous nerve typically lies in what muscle?

17. Regarding the anatomy of the axilla, pick one nerve (MCN, RAD, MED, ULN) for each:
    The nerve that passes though the coracobrachialis muscle: _____
    The nerve that passes between the axillary artery and vein: _____
    The nerve that follows the profunda brachii artery into the triceps muscle and spiral groove of the humerus: _____
    The nerve that passes from lateral to medial over the surface of the axillary artery and can be displaced to either side of the artery with probe compression: _____

18. True or False: In most subjects, the lateral femoral cutaneous nerve travels over (superficial to) the sartorius muscle near its insertion on the anterior superior iliac spine?

19. Which of the following statements regarding the femoral nerve are true? (Select all that apply.)
    A. The femoral nerve is always oval in shape.
    B. The femoral nerve is never triangular in shape.
    C. The femoral nerve can be triangular in shape, especially when imaged proximal to the inguinal ligament.

20. The femoral nerve lies deep to which of the following structure(s)? (Select all that apply.)
    A. Fascia lata
    B. Fascia iliaca
    C. Iliopsoas muscle
21. True or False: The saphenous nerve travels with the infrapatellar nerve and the nerve to the vastus medialis throughout most of its course in the thigh?
22. The saphenous nerve follows the course of what major structure as it descends the medial leg?
23. Which muscle separates the anterior and posterior divisions of the obturator nerve?
    A. Adductor longus
    B. Adductor magnus
    C. Adductor brevis
    D. Obturator internus
    E. Pectineus
24. Which adductor muscles are not innervated by the obturator nerve?
25. Name the blood vessel most closely associated with the following nerves:
    Saphenous nerve: _____
    Tibial nerve: _____
    Sural nerve: _____
    Superficial peroneal nerve: _____
    Deep peroneal nerve: _____

Answers to Text Questions

Answer 1: B

Clinical significance: Injection of a nonattenuating fluid into an attenuating sound field can cause enhancement of echoes deep to the fluid. This phenomenon is often seen during clinical blocks. Although this occurs after successful injections, fluid injected anywhere between the nerve and the skin surface will cause this effect.
Reference: Filly RA, Sommer FG, Minton MJ. Characterization of biological fluids by ultrasound and computed tomography. *Radiology.* 1980;134:167-171.

Answer 2: C

Clinical significance: Monofascicular nerves are more vulnerable to stretching and compression injury because they have a low connective tissue content.
References: Sunderland S. The connective tissues of peripheral nerves. *Brain.* 1965; 88:841-854.
Sunderland S, Bradley KC. The cross-sectional area of peripheral nerve trunks devoted to nerve fibers. *Brain.* 1949;72:428-449.
Sunderland S, Bradley KC. The perineurium of peripheral nerves. *Anat Rec.* 1952; 113:125-141.

Answer 3: A

Clinical significance: Nerves can be imaged at low frequencies (<10 MHz), but they appear as cordlike structures without internal fascicular architecture.
Reference: Giovagnorio F, Martinoli C. Sonography of the cervical vagus nerve: normal appearance and abnormal findings. *AJR Am J Roentgenol.* 2001;176:745-749.

Answer 4: C

Clinical significance: Probe compression is usually a quick and easy way to identify vascular structures. Compression tests are often useful for peripheral imaging.

Answer 5: B

Clinical significance: Anisotropy is a well-described property of many anatomic structures, including nerves and tendons.
References: Connolly DJ, Berman L, McNally EG. The use of beam angulation to overcome anisotropy when viewing human tendon with high frequency linear array ultrasound. *Br J Radiol.* 2001;74:183-185.
Soong J, Schafhalter-Zoppoth I, Gray AT. The importance of transducer angle to ultrasound visibility of the femoral nerve. *Reg Anesth Pain Med.* 2005;30:505.

Answer 6: C

Clinical significance: With experience, practitioners learn to manipulate the ultrasound transducer to enhance the received echoes from peripheral nerves.
Reference: Crass JR, van de Vegte GL, Harkavy LA. Tendon echogenicity: ex vivo study. *Radiology.* 1988;167:499-501.

Answer 7: A, B, C

Clinical significance: Needle tip visibility is crucial to real-time ultrasound guidance of all interventional procedures. Note that the cut of the bevel angle (D) has been studied and shown not to influence needle tip visibility.

References: Bondestam S, Kreula J. Needle tip echogenicity: a study with real-time ultrasound. *Invest Radiol.* 1989;24:555-560.

Hopkins RE, Bradley M: In vitro visualization of biopsy needles with ultrasound: a comparative study of standard and echogenic needles using an ultrasound phantom. *Clin Radiol.* 2001;56:499-502.

Schafhalter-Zoppoth I, McCulloch CE, Gray AT. Ultrasound visibility of needles used for regional nerve block: an in vitro study. *Reg Anesth Pain Med.* 2004;29:480-488.

Answer 8: C

Clinical significance: Distinguishing pleura from other nearby structures is crucial for interventional procedures in the supraclavicular region.

References: Ziskin MC, Thickman DI, Goldenberg NJ, et al. The comet tail artifact. *J Ultrasound Med.* 1982;1:1-7.

Thickman DI, Ziskin MC, Goldenberg NJ, Linder BE. Clinical manifestations of the comet tail artifact. *J Ultrasound Med.* 1983;2:225-230.

Answer 9: C

Reference: Han S, Medige J, Davis J, et al. Ultrasound velocity and broadband attenuation as predictors of load-bearing capacities of human calcanei. *Calcif Tissue Int.* 1997;60:21-25.

Answer 10: B

Clinical significance: Phrenic nerve block is often observed after brachial plexus block procedures in the neck. The phrenic nerve and the brachial plexus lie under the prevertebral fascia, which promotes the distribution of local anesthetic to both.

Reference: Kessler J, Schafhalter-Zoppoth I, Gray AT. An ultrasound study of the phrenic nerve in the posterior cervical triangle: implications for the interscalene brachial plexus block. *Reg Anesth Pain Med.* 2008;33:545-550.

Answer 11: C

Clinical significance: Distinguishing the first rib and pleura is critical during supraclavicular blocks. Like other bones, the first rib efficiently absorbs sound waves. Lung sliding and comet-tail artifact from reverberation are characteristics of the pleural line.

Reference: Thickman DI, Ziskin MC, Goldenberg NJ, Linder BE. Clinical manifestations of the comet tail artifact. *J Ultrasound Med.* 1983;2:225-230.

Answer 12: B

Clinical significance: The C5 and C6 ventral rami often travel over or through the anterior scalene muscle (5%-15% incidence). A cervical rib is an anatomic variant that occurs in 0.5% of the general population.

References: Harry WG, Bennett JD, Guha SC. Scalene muscles and the brachial plexus: Anatomical variations and their clinical significance. *Clin Anat.* 1997;10:250-252.

Mangrulkar VH, Cohen HL, Dougherty D. Sonography for diagnosis of cervical ribs in children. *J Ultrasound Med.* 2008;27:1083-1086.

Answer 13: The anterior scalene muscle

Clinical significance: (1) Diaphragmatic paralysis is an expected consequence of interscalene block (>99%). (2) Diaphragmatic contraction during electrolocation indicates anterior placement of the needle in relation to the brachial plexus.

Reference: Kessler J, Schafhalter-Zoppoth I, Gray AT. An ultrasound study of the phrenic nerve in the posterior cervical triangle: implications for the interscalene brachial plexus block. *Reg Anesth Pain Med.* 2008;33:545-550.

Answer 14: The second part of the axillary artery (under the pectoralis minor muscle)

Clinical significance: This is the anatomic position of the brachial plexus for infraclavicular block (posterior cord gives rise to the radial nerve, axillary nerve; medial cord gives rise to the median, ulnar, medial cutaneous nerves; lateral cord gives rise to the musculocutaneous, median).

Answer 15: Axillary and musculocutaneous nerves

Clinical significance: These nerves must be separately blocked when brachial plexus block is performed distal to the infraclavicular region.

Answer 16: The coracobrachialis

Clinical significance: The musculocutaneous nerve is not part of the neurovascular bundle in the axilla and therefore is frequently not anesthetized during conventional axillary blockade.

Answer 17

The nerve that passes though the coracobrachialis muscle: MCN
The nerve that passes between the axillary artery and vein: ULN
The nerve that follows the profunda brachii artery into the triceps: RAD
The nerve that passes from lateral to medial over the surface of the axillary artery and can be displaced to either side of the artery with probe compression: MED
Clinical significance: These characteristic features distinguish these peripheral nerves in the axilla.

Answer 18: True

Clinical significance: Ultrasound landmarks for regional block

Answer 19: C

Clinical significance: Identification of the femoral nerve is critical to block success. The femoral nerve typically lies in the groove between the iliacus and psoas muscles.
Reference: Gruber H, Peer S, Kovacs P, et al. The ultrasonographic appearance of the femoral nerve and cases of iatrogenic impairment. *J Ultrasound Med.* 2003;22:163-172.

Answer 20: A and B

Clinical significance: Needle tip placement in the correct layer is essential to femoral nerve block success.

Reference: Dalens B, Vanneuville G, Tanguy A. Comparison of the fascia iliaca compartment block with the 3-in-1 block in children. *Anesth Analg.* 1989;69:705-713.

Answer 21: True

Clinical significance: Concomitant block is likely. The infrapatellar nerve is usually considered a branch of the saphenous nerve.

Reference: Lundblad M, Kapral S, Marhofer P, Lonnqvist PA. Ultrasound-guided infrapatellar nerve block in human volunteers: description of a novel technique. *Br J Anaesth.* 2006; 97:710-714.

Answer 22: Saphenous vein

Clinical significance: The saphenous nerve is a sensory branch of femoral nerve. It innervates the medial leg. In most patients, the sensory block extends to the medial malleolus and medial foot, and in some patients, it extends to the great toe.

Reference: Benzon HT, Sharma S, Calimaran A. Comparison of the different approaches to saphenous nerve block. *Anesthesiology.* 2005;102:633-638.

Answer 23: C

Clinical significance: The adductor brevis is an important landmark for ultrasound-guided obturator nerve block.

Reference: Soong J, Schafhalter-Zoppoth I, Gray AT. Sonographic imaging of the obturator nerve for regional block. *Reg Anesth Pain Med.* 2007;32:146-151.

Answer 24: The pectineus (femoral nerve) and part of the adductor magnus (partially innervated by the sciatic nerve)

Clinical significance: Complete obturator block will reduce adduction strength (but not entirely).

Reference: Bouaziz H, Vial F, Jochum D, et al. An evaluation of the cutaneous distribution after obturator nerve block. *Anesth Analg.* 2002;94:445-449.

Answer 25

Saphenous nerve—saphenous vein

Tibial nerve—posterior tibial artery

Sural nerve—small saphenous vein

Superficial peroneal nerve—no major vessel is commonly associated (a small fibular artery is sometimes present)

Deep peroneal nerve—anterior tibial artery and dorsalis pedis artery

Clinical significance: Vascular landmarks often help identify peripheral nerves.

SELF-ASSESSMENT QUESTIONS: IMAGES

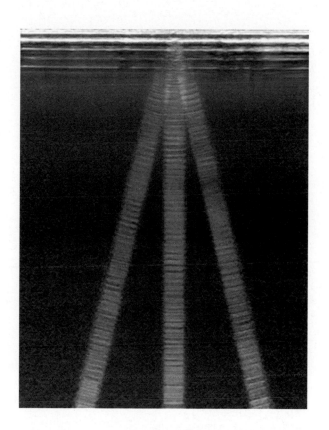

1. What does this linear array test tool image indicate?
   A. The ultrasound beam is of uniform width throughout the field.
   B. There are functional receiver apertures for three lines of sight.
   C. The dynamic focusing changes the test tool image as a function of displayed depth.
   D. There are three crystals in the array.

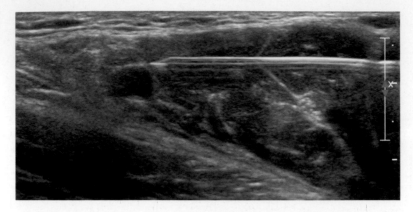

2. What term best describes the view of the nerve and needle approach shown here?
    A. Short-axis view of nerve, in-plane approach of needle
    B. Short-axis view of nerve, out-of-plane approach of needle
    C. Long-axis view of nerve, in-plane approach of needle
    D. Long-axis view of nerve, out-of-plane approach of needle

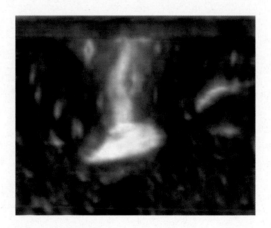

3. What does this image represent?
    A. Multiplanar reformatted (MPR) display
    B. Volume-rendered (VR) display
    C. Plane of acquisition display
    D. None of the above

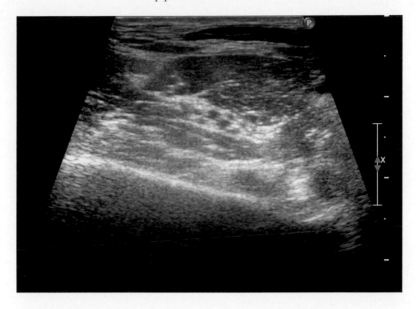

4. In this sonogram from the interscalene region, please identify the following:
   A. The phrenic nerve
   B. The brachial plexus
   C. The anterior scalene
   D. The middle scalene

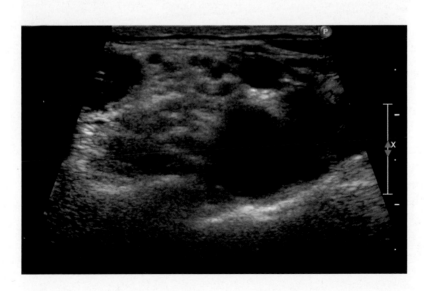

5. In this sonogram from the supraclavicular level, please identify the following:
   A. The subclavian artery
   B. The brachial plexus
   C. The first rib
   D. The pleura

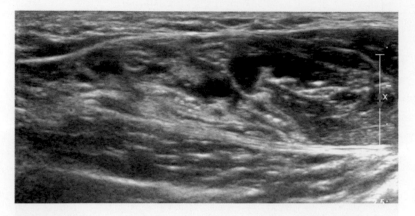

6. In this sonogram from the axilla after axillary block, please identify the following:
    A. The axillary artery
    B. The musculocutaneous nerve
    C. The median nerve
    D. The ulnar nerve
    E. The radial nerve

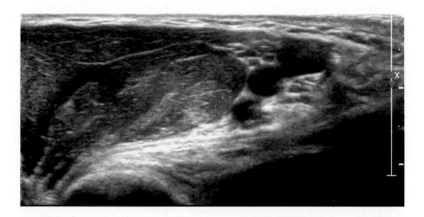

7. In this sonogram from the axilla, please identify the following:
    A. The musculocutaneous nerve
    B. The median nerve
    C. The ulnar nerve

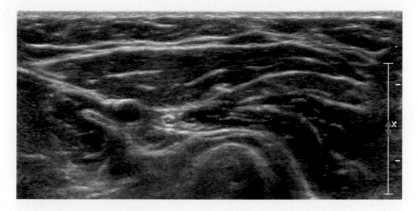

8. In this sonogram from the lateral forearm, please identify the following:
   A. The radial artery
   B. The superficial radial nerve
   C. The radius

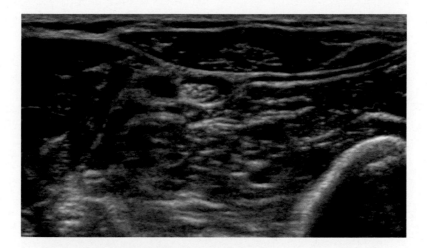

9. In this sonogram from the medial forearm, please identify the following:
   A. The ulnar artery
   B. The ulnar nerve
   C. The flexor carpi ulnaris tendon
   D. The ulna

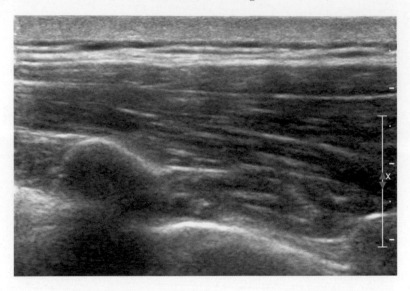

10. In this sonogram obtained during intercostal block, please identify the following:
    A. The ribs
    B. The pleural line

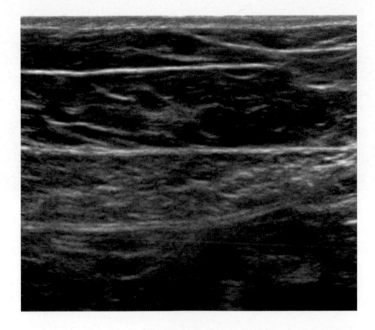

11. In this sonogram obtained during rectus sheath block, please identify the following:
    A. Rectus abdominis muscle
    B. The double layer

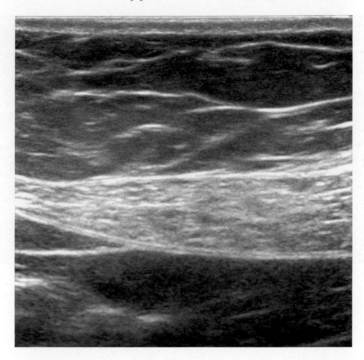

12. In this sonogram obtained during rectus sheath block, please identify the following:
    A. Linea semilunaris
    B. Rectus abdominis muscle
    C. Transversus abdominis muscle

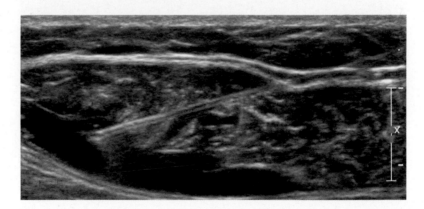

13. In this sonogram obtained during rectus sheath block, please identify the following:
    A. Rectus abdominis muscle
    B. The double layer
    C. Needle tip
    D. Local anesthetic distribution

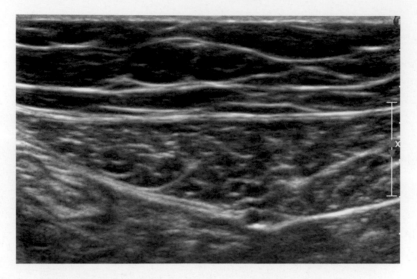

14. In this sonogram obtained during rectus sheath block, please identify the following:
    A. Rectus abdominis muscle
    B. The double layer
    C. Epigastric artery

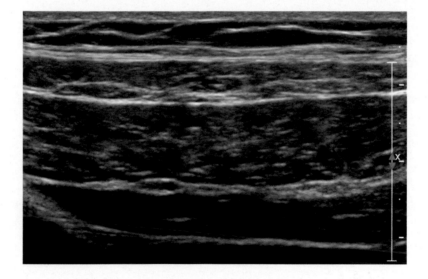

15. In this sonogram obtained during ilioinguinal block, please identify the following:
    A. External oblique
    B. Internal oblique
    C. Transversus
    D. Ilioinguinal nerves

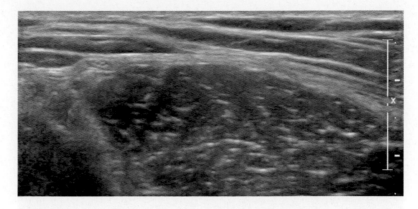

16. In this sonogram from the anterolateral thigh, please identify the following:
    A. The sartorius muscle
    B. The lateral femoral cutaneous nerve
    C. The fascia iliaca

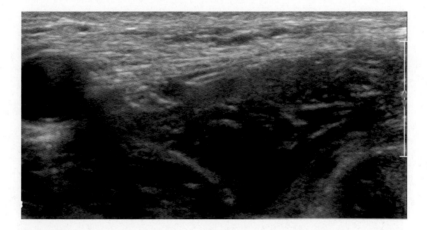

17. In this sonogram from the inguinal region, please identify the following:
    A. The femoral artery
    B. The femoral nerve
    C. The iliopsoas muscle
    D. The fascia iliaca
    E. The needle tip

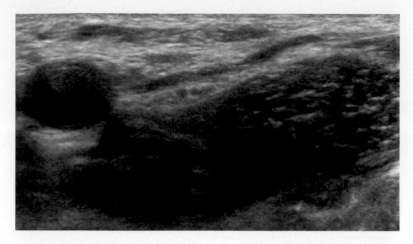

18. In this sonogram from the inguinal region, please identify the following:
    A. The femoral artery
    B. The femoral nerve
    C. The lateral circumflex femoral artery

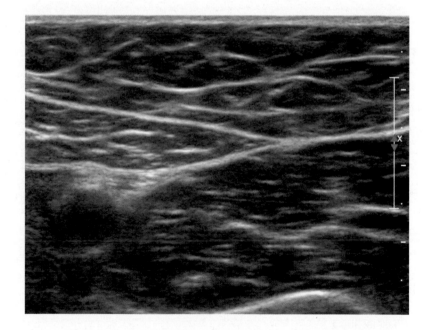

19. In this sonogram from the medial mid-thigh, please identify the following:
    A. The sartorius
    B. The vastus medialis
    C. Femoral artery
    D. Subsartorial plexus

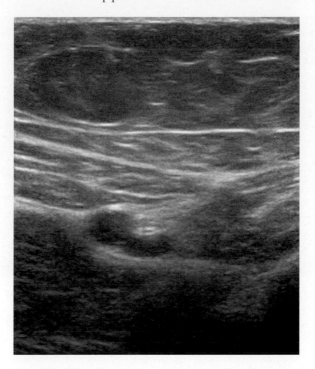

20. In this sonogram from the medial mid-thigh, please identify the following:
    A. The sartorius
    B. The vastus medialis
    C. Femoral artery
    D. Subsartorial plexus
    E. Femoral vein

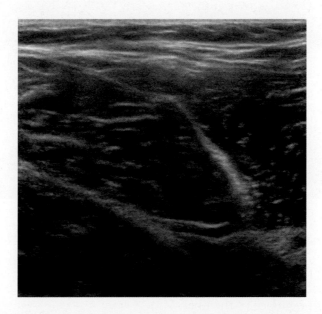

21. In this sonogram from the proximal medial thigh, please identify the following:
    A. The adductor brevis
    B. The anterior division of the obturator nerve
    C. The posterior division of the obturator nerve

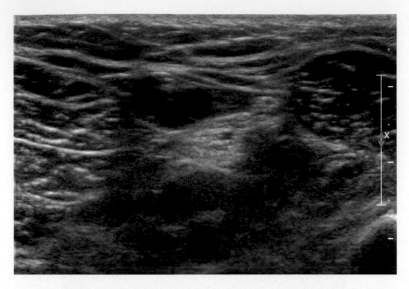

22. In this sonogram from the popliteal fossa, please identify the following:
    A. The common peroneal nerve
    B. The tibial nerve
    C. The popliteal artery
    D. The popliteal vein

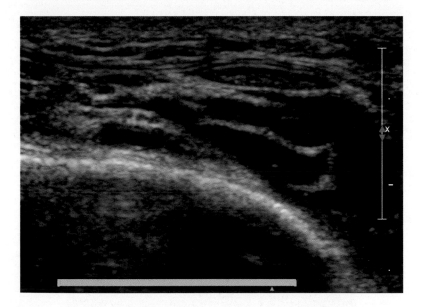

23. In this sonogram from the anterior leg proximal to the ankle, please identify the following:
    A. The deep peroneal nerve
    B. The anterior tibial artery
    C. The anterior surface of the tibia

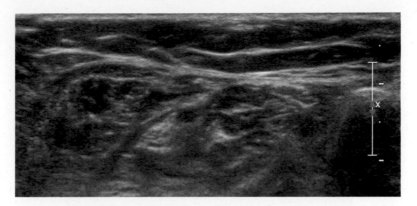

24. In this sonogram from the medial leg proximal to the ankle, please identify the following:
    A. The tibial artery
    B. The tibial nerve
    C. The flexor digitorum longus tendon
    D. The tibia

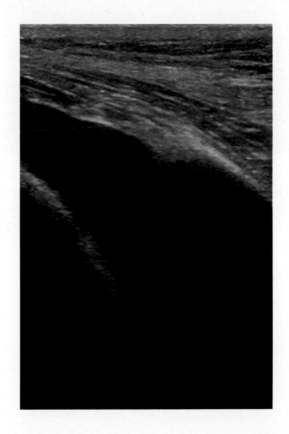

25. Which of the following is consistent with this sonogram from an intercostal interspace?
    A. Normal lung
    B. Pneumothorax
    C. Pleural effusion

Answers to Image Questions

Answer 1: B

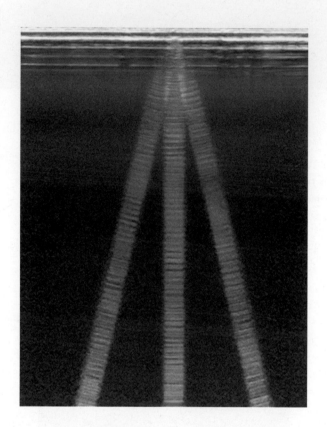

Clinical significance: The linear array test tool can be used to test for nonfunctioning elements and to determine how many lines of sight are used for spatial compound imaging.
Reference: Goldstein A, Ranney D, McLeary RD. Linear array test tool. *J Ultrasound Med.* 1989;8:385-397.

Answer 2: A

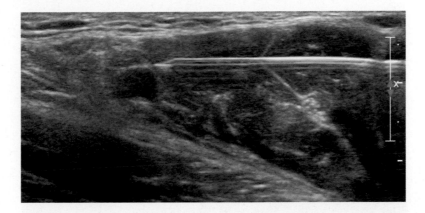

Clinical significance: Many approaches to regional block have been described. In clinical practice, short-axis views are most common.

Reference: Gray AT. Ultrasound-guided regional anesthesia: current state of the art. *Anesthesiology.* 2006;104:368-373.

Answer 3: B

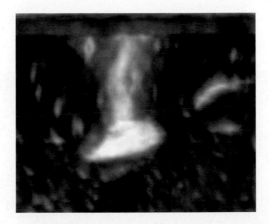

Reference: Rose SC, Nelson TR, Deutsch R. Display of 3-dimensional ultrasonographic images for interventional procedures: volume-rendered versus multiplanar display. *J Ultrasound Med.* 2004;23:1465-1473.

Answer 4: See labeled sonogram.

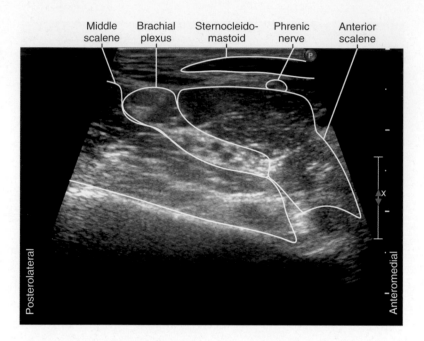

Clinical significance: Ultrasound landmarks for regional block

Answer 5: See labeled sonogram.

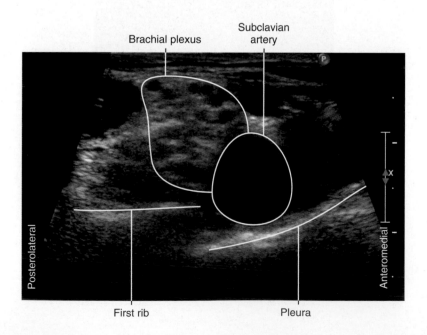

Clinical significance: Supraclavicular blocks carry an inherent risk for pneumothorax because of the proximity of pleura and brachial plexus. Differentiation of first rib and pleura is imperative • to help reduce the incidence of this complication.

Answer 6: See labeled sonogram.

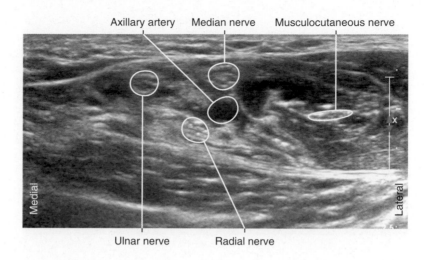

Clinical significance: Ultrasound landmarks for regional block

Answer 7: See labeled sonogram.

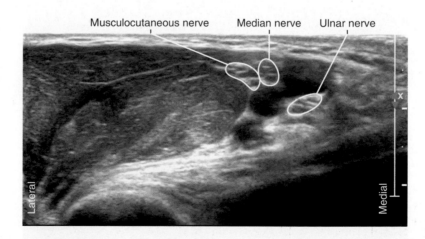

Clinical significance: In this example, the median nerve and musculocutaneous nerve are fused together (a low-lying lateral cord).

Answer 8: See labeled sonogram.

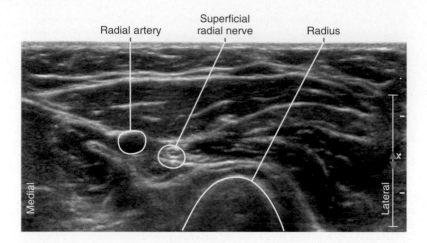

Clinical significance: Ultrasound landmarks for regional block. The superficial radial nerve joins and leaves the radial artery on the lateral side of the forearm.

Answer 9: See labeled sonogram.

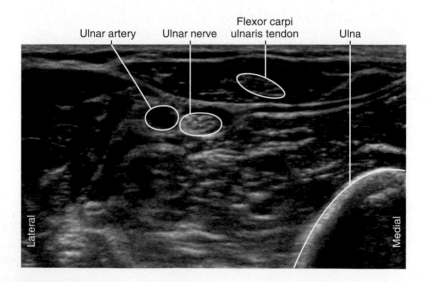

Clinical significance: Ultrasound landmarks for regional block. The ulnar nerve typically lies between the ulnar artery and the flexor carpi ulnaris tendon. In patients with superficial ulnar artery, this relation does not hold.

Answer 10: See labeled sonogram.

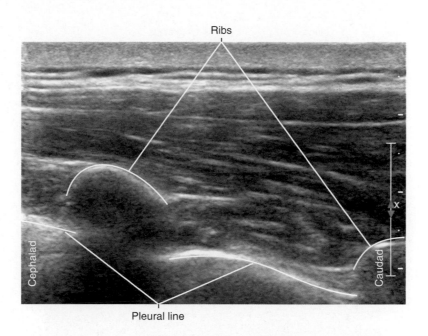

Clinical significance: Ultrasound landmarks for regional block. The pleura has a distinct bright appearance on ultrasound scans.

Answer 11: See labeled sonogram.

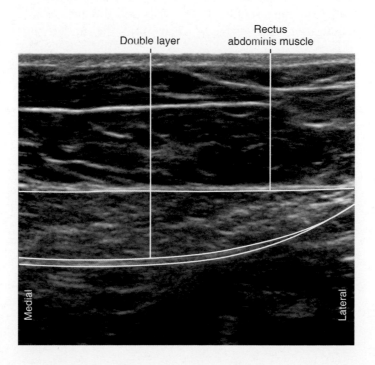

Clinical significance: Ultrasound landmarks for regional block. The double layer is composed of the transversalis fascia and transversus aponeurosis.

Answer 12: See labeled sonogram.

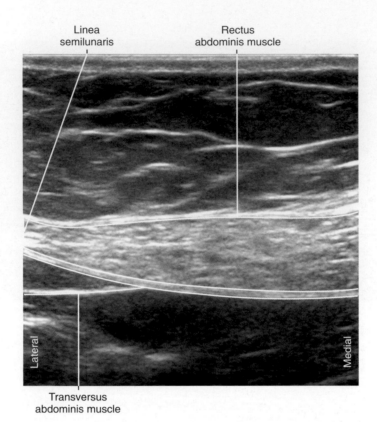

Clinical significance: Ultrasound landmarks for regional block. The extent of rectus sheath block is limited by the linea semilunaris laterally and the linea alba at the midline. In this case, the orientation of the image is clear from the underlying transversus muscle laterally.

Answer 13: See labeled sonogram.

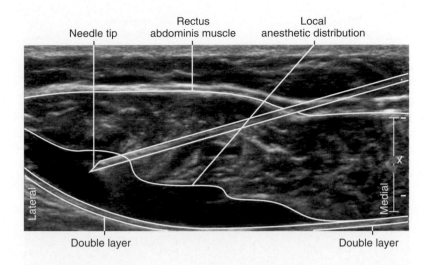

Clinical significance: Ultrasound landmarks for regional block. Rectus sheath injections should distribute between the rectus abdominis muscle and the double layer.

Answer 14: See labeled sonogram.

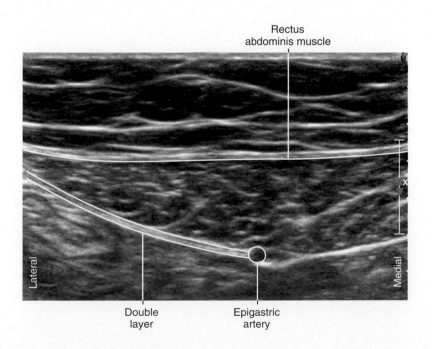

Clinical significance: Ultrasound landmarks for regional block. Epigastric arteries have a variable position within the rectus sheath.

Answer 15: See labeled sonogram.

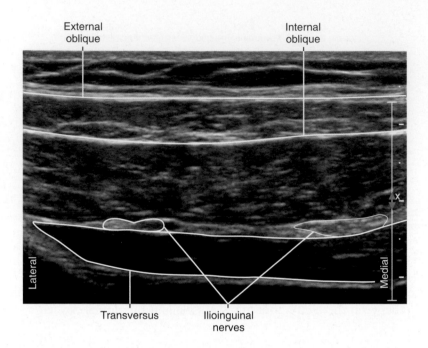

Clinical significance: Ultrasound landmarks for regional block. The ilioinguinal nerves are usually visualized between the internal oblique and transversus muscles of the lateral abdominal wall.

Reference: Eichenberger U, Greher M, Kirchmair L, et al. Ultrasound-guided blocks of the ilioinguinal and iliohypogastric nerve: accuracy of a selective new technique confirmed by anatomical dissection. *Br J Anaesth.* 2006;97:238-243.

Answer 16: See labeled sonogram.

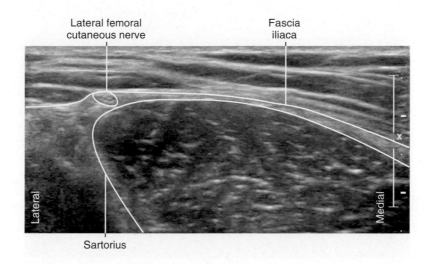

Clinical significance: Ultrasound landmarks for regional block

Answer 17: See labeled sonogram.

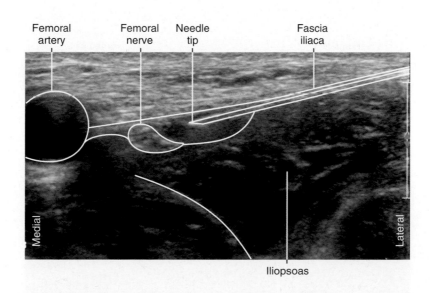

Clinical significance: Ultrasound landmarks for regional block
References: Gruber H, Peer S, Kovacs P, et al. The ultrasonographic appearance of the femoral nerve and cases of iatrogenic impairment. *J Ultrasound Med.* 2003;22:163-272.
Dalens B, Vanneuville G, Tanguy A. Comparison of the fascia iliaca compartment block with the 3-in-1 block in children. *Anesth Analg.* 1989;69:705-713.

Answer 18: See labeled sonogram.

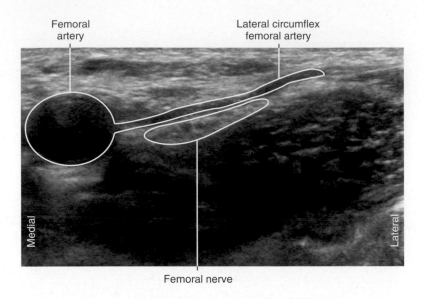

Clinical significance: Ultrasound landmarks for regional block. The lateral circumflex femoral artery is a branch of the femoral artery that overlies the femoral nerve.

Answer 19: See labeled sonogram.

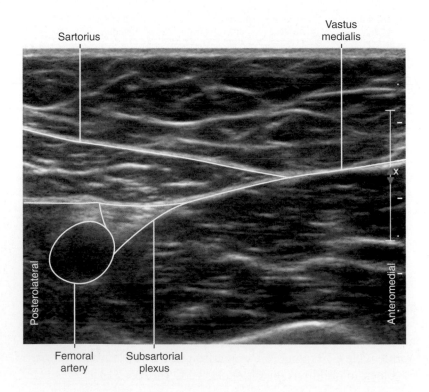

Clinical significance: Ultrasound landmarks for regional block

Answer 20: See labeled sonogram.

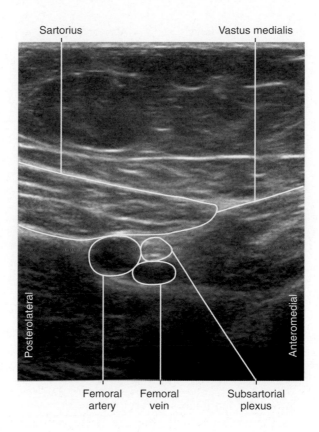

Clinical significance: Ultrasound landmarks for regional block. In this case, light touch with the transducer reveals the femoral vein under the artery and nerves.

Answer 21: See labeled sonogram.

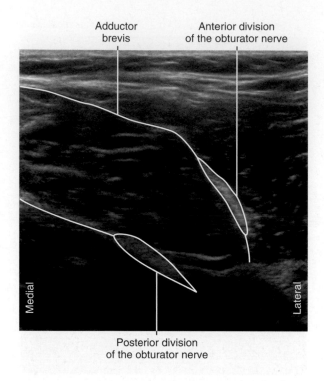

Clinical significance: Ultrasound landmarks for regional block

Reference: Soong J, Schafhalter-Zoppoth I, Gray AT. Sonographic imaging of the obturator nerve for regional block. *Reg Anesth Pain Med.* 2007;32:146-151.

Answer 22: See labeled sonogram.

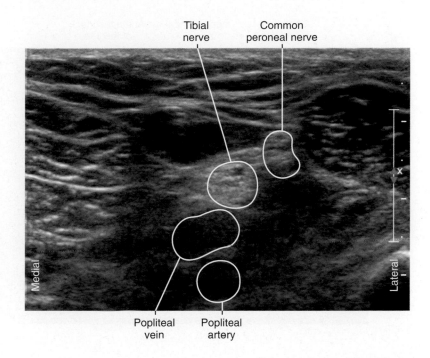

Clinical significance: The common peroneal nerve has about half the cross-sectional area of the tibial nerve. The common peroneal nerve lies lateral and posterior to the tibial nerve in the popliteal fossa.

Reference: Heinemeyer O, Reimers CD. Ultrasound of radial, ulnar, median, and sciatic nerves in healthy subjects and patients with hereditary motor and sensory neuropathies. *Ultrasound Med Biol.* 1999;25:481-485.

Answer 23: See labeled sonogram.

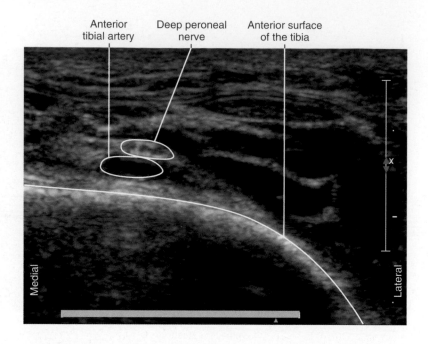

Clinical significance: The deep peroneal nerve characteristically crosses over the anterior tibial artery proximal to the ankle.

Answer 24: See labeled sonogram.

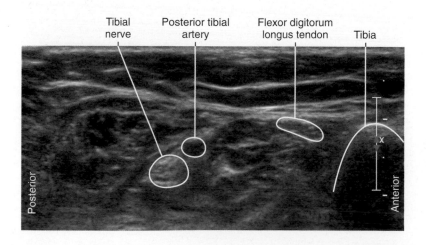

Clinical significance: Ultrasound landmarks for regional block. The tibial nerve lies on the heel side of the tibial artery. The flexor digitorum longus tendon lies closer to the tibia than the tibial nerve.

Answer 25: C

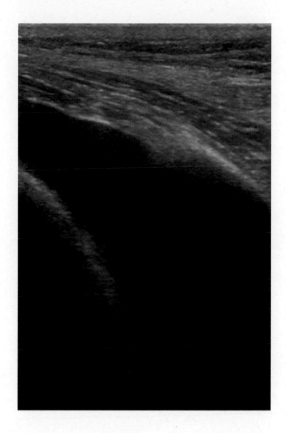

Clinical significance: In this example, a large pleural effusion lies over the lung surface. The image demonstrates chest pathology that can be detected with ultrasound imaging.

INDEX

Note: Page numbers followed by b, f, and t indicate boxes, figures, and tables, respectively.